Final Weight LOSS

Lose Weight • Celebrate Your Life • Never Be Overweight Again

by

Jase Simmons

To Sean ~ Enjoy in great health. Jase Simmons

FINAL WEIGHT LOSS
Lose Weight • Celebrate Your Life •
Never Be Overweight Again

Copyright © 2013 by Jase Simmons

Book Design
Amy Livingstone, Sacred Art Studio
www.sacredartstudio.net

ISBN-13: 978-0615748672
ISBN-10: 0615748678

DEDICATION

This book is dedicated to all those who gave me the courage to choose an exceptional path in search of a greater quality of life.

TABLE OF CONTENTS

INTRODUCTION

Five weeks from my 43rd birthday, I weighed 271 pounds. Because I'm 5'10", that meant that I was not just overweight, I was obese. I had already tried every gimmicky weight-loss program I could get my hands on. None of them worked. My desperation led me to create the self-designed weight-loss program you'll find in this book. I began using it on April 25, 2011 and it has altered the course of my life forever.

My weight-loss goal had nothing to do with losing a specific amount of weight and everything to do with staying on my program. As you can see, the results speak for themselves. I lost 83 pounds by the end of calendar year 2011. I celebrated the one-year anniversary of my final weight loss (April 25, 2012) weighing 176 pounds—that's 95 pounds lost. I turned 44 on May 31, 2012, weighing 170 pounds—101 pounds lost!

I am certain that anyone can apply the weight-loss program I created for myself. It is convenient, efficient, effective, and easy to understand. I am now someone whose happiness in life will never be compromised again due to his weight problem.

When I was obese, I believed that I had been born with a much slower resting metabolic rate than most people I knew—my body just didn't burn calories that easily. This belief was my justification for being overweight for most of my adult life. I felt hopeless. I often compared myself to some of my close friends who seemed to have miracle metabolisms—regardless of what they ate or how little they exercised, they never gained any weight.

I have other friends that exercise occasionally and eat whatever they want who have never been overweight. Most people I know don't do any challenging exercise, eat whatever they want, and comfortably walk around carrying an extra 15-20 pounds. During my obese life, I desperately wanted to be in this group. Unfortunately, I did not fall into any of these groups. There seemed to be no upside limit to how much weight I could gain.

In the next pages, you'll read the story of all of my weight frustrations. You will probably be able to relate to some or all of my challenges. My obesity story isn't anything special. In fact, according to the most recent obesity statistics, more than two-thirds of all adults in the United States are overweight and over one-third are obese. One-third of all children and adolescents in the United States are overweight and more than 15% are obese. It is projected that by 2030, 86% of all people in the United States will be overweight and 42% will be obese. I didn't want to be one of those people. You don't have to be one either.

If you are ready to give yourself a life rather than a life sentence, I am ready to help you. I was successful in identifying the source of my never-ending weight problems and I turned my health around before it was too late. I look forward to helping you do the same!

TRACKING MY WEIGHT LOSS

Date	Milestone	Weight in Pounds
2011		
April 25	Start final weight loss/Start Master Cleanse	271
May 9	Come off Master Cleanse	248
July 25	Three months into program: down 52 pounds	219
August 25	Dropped below 210	209
September 23	Down 70 pounds	201
September 28	Below 200 pounds for the first time this century	198.5
December 9	Left for Hawaii to run the Honolulu Marathon	194
December 23	Below 190 pounds for the first time in 15 years	189.5
January 1	Happy New Year	188
2012		
March 13	Undergo back surgery for herniated disk (suspend exercise other than walking for 2 months)	181
April 6	Below 180 Pounds for the first time in 20 years	179
April 25	Happy One-Year Weight-Loss Anniversary (95 pounds lost)	176
May 13	Resume moderate exercise	171
May 31	Turned 44: 101 pounds lost	170
Summer/Fall	Weight loss ends and weight stabilizes	167-170

Chapter ONE

MY STORY

In April 2011, I was in San Francisco on business. I was getting ready to play a round of golf with one of my clients. Typical of the climate in San Francisco, it was much cooler and windier than I had anticipated and I hadn't brought the right kind of golf jacket with me. So I went into the pro shop and tried on what I thought was a size 2XL. I could barely get it on and it was very uncomfortable. I was certain that I had accidentally put on a size XL by mistake. When I took off the jacket and glanced at the tag, it was a 2XL. This was the moment that my obesity and all of the adversarial effects it was having on my life became real. My life wasn't being inconvenienced by my weight problem, it was being ruined by my weight problem.

I could not believe I had just entered the world of not being able to walk into a department store, golf shop, or other clothing store and buy a garment off the rack. With few exceptions, most clothing stores don't offer clothing in 3XL sizes.

A few days later, April 22 to be exact, my wife Lisa and I were at Creswell Coffee, a great local café we visit most mornings. Having arrived home from San Francisco and weighed myself, I learned the painful truth—I weighed 271 pounds. I was within 5 pounds of being the most overweight that I had ever been. The time had come for me to have a very serious conversation with Lisa. I needed to ask her to support me in what I was about to do: start a self-designed weight-loss program the following Monday.

My weight had spiraled out of control

I fought my weight for 27 of the first 42 years of my life. I had given up on the idea that I was ever going to be thin quite a while before. Specifically, it was when Lisa and I returned home from our honeymoon in April 2004. I weighed 258 pounds three months before we got married and knew I needed to lose weight quickly. I didn't want to be the most overweight person at my wedding, especially since we were getting married on the Big Island of Hawaii. Over the next three months, I managed to lose 41 pounds and arrived in Hawaii for the wedding festivities weighing 217 pounds, still overweight but far better than 258 pounds. I had lost that weight by putting myself in a weight-loss boot-camp situation.

I enjoyed our honeymoon and did not make my diet or weight loss the focus of our trip. We spent the first week in Kauai followed by three days in Las Vegas. When we returned to Oregon, I went to the gym to resume my pre-wedding exercise program.

Before my workout that day, I got on the scale at the gym, the same scale I weighed myself on each day before we left for Hawaii. I was certain that I had gained a few pounds while we were gone because I'd indulged myself during most meals and ate large amounts of whatever I wanted, mostly highly processed foods. Although I was not eating properly, I exercised most days while we were away. I also body-surfed in the ocean and went on a few hikes.

I was prepared for the scale to reveal that I had gained four or five pounds but that wasn't what it showed. **I had gained 14 pounds!** I would have understood 14 pounds if I'd spent the previous ten days eating 5,000 calories a day of ice cream sandwiches. Instead, although I knew I had eaten heartily and enjoyed my fair share of cocktails—it was my wedding and my honeymoon, after all—I had still been physically active!

The scale wasn't lying: I was 14 pounds heavier than I had been before Lisa and I left for Hawaii to get married. I was distraught and immediately exited the gym. What was the point of exercising? I resigned myself to being overweight for the rest of my life.

I consistently gained significant amounts of weight and intermittently lost very little during the next seven years. I looked in the mirror and often shook my head, always arriving at the conclusion that there was simply nothing that could be done. I was convinced that I was snake-bit with a sorry metabolism and would always be overweight. I learned to live a compromised life as an overweight and then obese person.

Here are some of the compromises I lived with as an obese person:

- I wore large, bulky clothing to hide my body frame. I frequently dressed inappropriately to hide my obesity, particularly in the summer by wearing bulky sports jackets regardless of the temperature. I wore golf jackets when it was blistering hot outside without a cloud in the sky. Although my skin felt like asphalt melting in the desert, I was too embarrassed to play golf in a short-sleeve shirt.
- I rarely wore button-down shirts. The one exception was my "stylish for the fat guy" Tommy Bahama shirt (size 2XL) untucked over a pair of baggy Tommy Hilfiger Slacks. God Bless those Tommy Hilfiger slacks—they stretch like spandex on crack!
- I wore nice sports coats only when forced to and never wore a tie. When I wore a tie, I looked like my neck had just swallowed my face.
- I avoided having my picture taken whenever possible. If I was forced to be in a picture, I stood behind my wife with my arms wrapped around the front of her waist. Lisa is an inch and a half shorter than I am—when I stood behind her, the picture revealed my large face and bald head while hiding most of my enormous stomach and thick neck, legs, and torso.

There were many events that should have been a weight-loss wake-up call for me. Here are a few examples:

- I knew I weighed more than 250 pounds and refused to get on the scale anymore.
- I reached the end of the strap on a normal airplane seatbelt. Had I gained a few additional pounds, it would have been seat-belt extension time for me. In addition, I watched people grimace when they realized they would be sitting next to me on a plane flight.
- I used to limp and cramp each time I played 18 holes of golf. I convinced myself that my pain was due to the fact that I was getting older and my body did not work the way it used to—a garbage excuse given that I had played golf with men who were nearly twice my age who were neither limping nor cramping after their golf round.
- I woke up one night and felt my left arm tingling. Lisa drove me to the emergency room. During my examination, the doctor diplomatically asked me what I was doing for exercise to try to stay in shape. I told him I played golf. The doctor smiled, I smiled, and Lisa even smiled. The doctor immediately informed me (as if I didn't know) that golf was not keeping my weight down and encouraged me to join a gym and commit to a regular exercise program. For the record, my heart was fine. I would have had only myself to blame if it had not been.

For a long time, I lived a weight-compromised life and my whole life was a struggle because I was so overweight. Then I went to San Francisco and walked into that golf shop and couldn't find a jacket that fit me. That was the last straw!

Had it really come to this? Was my weight ever going to plateau? Was I really headed down the path of type II diabetes and living with the daily drug regimen that accompanies this condition? Would I have to start wearing tennis shoes with springs attached to the heels? Was I ready to give up golf?

I returned home from San Francisco angry—angry at myself for being so obese. I was tired of blaming my age and my metabolism for my weight problem. I decided to take a good look in the mirror. I was never going to lose weight until I was honest with myself about the fact that being obese was due to my own living habits. The time was now for me to stop making excuses and start solving my problem!

The coffee shop on April 22, 2011

Lisa and I have a wonderful marriage and I love her more than anything in this world. That day, I looked into her eyes while talking to her and knew that despite how happy we were, I felt sorry for her. She was married to someone who was obese. Due to my living habits and lame excuses, she was on her way to being a widow at a young age. It was my fault, not her fault. The reality of this was much worse than the golf jacket incident I had just experienced a couple of days earlier.

I asked Lisa to support me in losing weight. She had supported me before, but all of my former attempts to lose weight had been failures—I always regained the weight I had lost and added more weight. She readily agreed to support me. I knew I was not going to fail this time! I was not simply going to lose weight; I was going to travel all the way to the opposite side of the world from being overweight and never return.

My plan

My plan was to start my final weight-loss effort on Monday, April 25, 2011, with a two- week cleanse. I spent the weekend conceptualizing a permanent healthy eating and consistent exercise program that I would implement immediately following the cleanse. I knew my program would need to be one that I would not only use for weight loss, but one I could continue to follow for the rest of my life.

My current eating plan consisted of eating whatever I wanted (highly processed foods including fast food and junk food) in huge quantities, drinking whatever I wanted (soda, milkshakes, coffee, beer, cocktails, wine, etc.) in huge volume, and refusing to do any consistent and meaningful form of exercise.

I would wake up and decide I was too busy to exercise. Then I'd eat an unhealthy convenience breakfast: a coffee drink filled with artificial sweetener while consuming a breakfast sandwich loaded with processed ingredients. I'd eat another convenient, highly processed nutrient-poor meal for lunch to satisfy my starvation. I'd eat yet another nutrient-poor meal for dinner and promise myself that I would begin my real weight loss the following day. I'd wake up the next day, weigh myself, and realize that I had gained weight the day before, a day in which I was supposed to start losing weight. So I'd decide to put off losing weight until the following week. Ultimately the following week became the following month. The following month became the following year. The following year became size 3XL golf jacket time.

Before starting the cleanse, I completed a self-analysis and arrived at the very real understanding of what had actually transpired to get me to 271 pounds. I made peace with that and decided that I was only going to look forward and not back with regrets. During that weekend, I addressed all of my issues related to diet, exercise, and weight loss. I decided that my weight problem **was not** because I didn't have enough time to eat right and exercise—that was an excuse. I decided I would no longer sacrifice my health and fall back into the following vicious weight-gain cycle.

HOW I USED TO EAT

BREAKFAST

Option 1:
Go to a coffee shop and order a bagel, pastry, or breakfast sandwich and down it with a 16 oz. latte with added processed sweetener.

Option 2:
Have a breakfast meeting with a client and order steak and eggs. Eat the steak and eggs with a side of toast (sourdough for me), hash browns, and juice refilled multiple times throughout the meal.

Option 3:
Skip breakfast and prepare to eat like a starving elephant at lunch.

LUNCH

Option 1:
Dine at any convenience restaurant that would service my food-craving choice of the day and eat as much as possible.

Option 2:
Dine at a nice restaurant and order one of the many tasty yet unhealthy highly processed entrée choices on the menu. Eat as much hot, buttered bread before the meal as politely possible. Eat my entire entrée and make the plate look like it was just removed clean from a commercial dishwasher.

DINNER

Option 1:
Bring home a take-out meal from a fancy-sounding place that serves flavorful highly processed food loaded with sugar and salt (we don't cook much at our house).

Option 2:
Go out to dinner. Eat at a fine dining establishment and choose one of the many tasty yet unhealthy options on the menu. Eat as much hot, buttered bread before the meal as politely possible. Eat the entire entrée and make the plate look like it was just removed clean from a commercial dishwasher. Eat a shared dessert with the table.

SNACK TIME

Eat anything I desired multiple times throughout the day whether I was hungry or not.

Summary of My Self-Analysis

- I completely gave up on myself when I stepped on the scale at the gym after returning home from our honeymoon in April 2004.
- I was addicted to highly processed foods loaded with chemicals and preservatives.
- I drank very little water—many days the only water I consumed was the melted ice in my diet soda or cocktail glass.
- Although it is possible that I was born with a slower metabolism than most people, the real truth is I did no meaningful exercise. My only exercise included practicing and playing golf.
- When I started a workout program at a health club, I never stuck with it.
- I did not dedicate any time to my own physical fitness, health, and well-being.
- I joined health clubs, signed up for training sessions, and never stuck with them. I "intended" to get back to it but I never committed to any exercise program long enough to make any difference.

During my self-analysis weekend, I arrived at the conclusion that I needed to change my lifestyle if I was to conquer my weight problem for good.

The Obvious Solutions

- Complete a healthy cleanse and eliminate as many toxins as possible that had accumulated in my body for years as a result of my poor diet.
- Create a convenient, permanent healthy-eating program that I would be able to adhere to following the cleanse in order to continue to lose weight and keep it off permanently.
- Commit to a weekly exercise program.

The Next Chapter

In the next chapter, you will have an opportunity to do your own reality check. Before we can fully commit to losing weight permanently, I believe we must be completely honest with ourselves. You must make peace with how you arrived at your present situation just as I did.

Chapter TWO

YOUR STORY

Reality Check for the Overweight/Obese Person

Being overweight has compromised your life in ways that you are and are not aware of. You wake up every day, look in the mirror, and feel disgusted. You wonder why you don't have a metabolism like other people you know, one that will allow you to stay thin despite your poor eating habits and minimal exercise activity. You have convinced yourself that you do not have the time to commit to a consistent exercise program that will make any meaningful difference in your life. You've tried many diets that promised you the world but really only offered temporary solutions that were never sustainable and made you miserable. If you were to accurately describe your present situation, you would acknowledge the following:

- You feel like you are so overweight that even if you decided to adopt a healthier way of living, it would take too long and would not make a significant difference in your life.
- You feel like you have "more important" things going on right now and do not have time to make changes in your life.
- You don't have the desire or inclination to join a health club or go to the health club you currently pay for each month and commit to an exercise program because you find it boring. You would rather spend your free time engaging in a hobby that does not require any physical dedication.
- You believe you will ultimately take care of your weight problem in the future and don't need to deal with it right now.

You have adopted poor eating habits and have no idea that you are probably addicted to highly processed foods that contain excessive amounts of empty calories: simple carbohydrates, sugars, additives, and man-made chemicals and preservatives that provide your body with little or no nutrition. You are constantly hungry and fight food cravings every day.

You mostly eat foods that contain few or no nutrients. You are unaware that most of the so-called healthy snacks you consume are processed food bombs loaded with simple carbs, simple sugars, and chemicals that keep you in the vicious cycle of constantly craving more food. You dream about what it would be like to not be overweight, but you cannot imagine waking up and starting your day without processed carbs, simple sugars, and caffeine drinks filled with artificial sweeteners. You are convinced that your body actually needs these things for you to function on a meaningful level throughout your day. You are unhappy at work or unhappy at home (or both) and eat for pleasure rather than to nourish your body or fuel your exercise.

I have been there! Until I admitted to all of these facts and got honest with myself, I knew that change was not possible. Assuming you are overweight, you must accept that most if not all of what you have just read applies to you. Your future weight loss will only become a reality if you are completely honest about your present situation. I am not telling you to assign blame; I am insisting that you acknowledge the truth of your life and your current relationship to food and exercise.

If you can do that, you are on your way to deciding that the condition of being overweight, out of shape, and fighting food addictions has severely compromised your life, and you are ready to commit to a healthy way of living in order to lose all of your excess weight and keep it off forever.

Acknowledging that you need to make a change in your life means that you have accepted the fact that you are not one of the fortunate few who can eat whatever they want, do little or no meaningful exercise, and be someone who is not overweight. You have accepted that your search for the magic diet pill or supplement that will enable you to miraculously lose all of your excess weight while allowing you to continue living the unhealthy lifestyle you have become accustomed to does not exist. There isn't one, I promise! I would have found it myself if it existed.

The reality check you have just completed may not be easy to accept. Mine wasn't and I empathize with you.

The Mental Aspect of Changing Your Life to Lose Weight

Most people resist making incidental changes in their life even if it affords them the opportunity for an incredible life upgrade. Everyone automatically assumes that the concept of change involves taking a risk. This aspect alone prevents most people from succeeding at permanent weight loss.

Take a step back and analyze what I have just written from a perspective other than weight loss for a minute. How many times have you ended a toxic personal relationship at "just the right time" instead of sticking around way too damn long until you were finally forced to walk away in order to preserve what little sanity you had left?

Now analyze your relationship with being overweight from the same perspective. You are at a crossroad in your life. Do you want to be the permanent client of a weight-loss clinic? Do you want to pay for and take prescription medications every day to counteract the adverse effects of being overweight? Do you want to continue to stand on the sidelines and watch other people enjoy what you wish you could do if you were not overweight or obese? Or, are you ready to upgrade your life?

In the last year of speaking publicly about my experience, overweight people have asked me how I was losing so much weight because they desperately wanted to lose their weight too. When I described the weight-loss program I created for myself, many would interject and start telling me what they "could not do" related to diet and exercise because they were not able to imagine themselves doing it. I understood where they were coming from. I had been there for a long time.

Most of the time when we say "I can't" what we are really saying is "I won't," which really means "I am not willing to." For a long time, I was not willing to either. But then I got to a different place. I had another "aha" moment and this time I really listened. From that moment on, I was able to accept that I needed to make dramatic changes if I wanted things to be different. Would it be easy? Probably not. Would it be worth it? Absolutely! What the hell did I have to lose anyway? My life was already being ruined as a result of my obesity!

From this moment forward, you need to accept that your attitude toward diet and exercise must change dramatically if you want to lose weight permanently. You do not have to deprive yourself on my weight-loss program! You will live differently so that you can live a better life, which will give you every opportunity from a health and wellness perspective to live a longer life.

You must be open to all recommendations. Do not pre-suppose that you will be unable to follow my program simply because you cannot imagine yourself doing it! You must think like a winner from day one when you begin your final weight loss. Weight loss will only be the beginning of much greater things to come your way when you take control of your life.

Setting a Goal

The only goal I set when I started my program was to stick with it, and that is the only goal you will need. Stick with my program and your weight will come off. Unlike many other weight-loss programs, I encourage you to get on the scale and weigh yourself every morning—weigh yourself immediately after you wake up and use the bathroom. You will be amazed by how much weight you are losing.

Do not set a weight-loss goal. When I lost 95 pounds last year, I **never** set a goal of how much weight I planned to lose. I encourage you not to choose a maximum amount of weight you want to lose either. Why put unnecessary pressure on yourself? Why limit yourself?

Before my weight loss, I could not have imagined that I would ever weigh less than 200 pounds again, yet after a year I weighed 176 pounds, and when I turned 44 five weeks later, I weighed 170 pounds. Since then, my weight has fluctuated between 167 and 171 pounds.

Your body will ultimately find its most appropriate weight once you are living a healthier life. Analyze this concept another way. Your body spent years constantly adjusting to your heavier weight based on your unhealthy lifestyle. Rest assured, it will gravitate down and find its healthiest weight when you give it a chance!

Weight Fluctuations

There will be days when your body is assimilating everything (including your strength-training exercises). Occasionally the scale may reveal that you have stayed the same weight or gained a pound from one day to the next. This is not an issue and you should not get discouraged! You will experience weight loss consistently on my program until you have lost all of the weight you need to lose.

Muscle weighs more than fat. You will gain muscle while losing fat on my weight-loss program just like I did. There were many occasions during the last year when the scale did not reveal that I had lost any weight for two or three days in a row and then it would display a loss of as much as two pounds per day on consecutive days thereafter.

Your Reward

Your reward is directly correlated to your weight loss. Once you have completed the first three weeks on my weight-loss program, you can start dreaming about how you are going to reward yourself once you have lost all of the weight you need to lose. You will not only have lost a substantial amount of weight during the first three weeks on my program, you will have made a commitment to living a much healthier life. You will be physically and mentally feeling all of the benefits of consuming a healthy diet. You will be amazed by how much your fitness levels have improved in such a short time and you will be able to realistically start to dream about enjoying some of life's greatest activities that you never thought would be possible.

When you start to conceptualize your reward, dream big! Mentally, your outlook will be different. You might choose to engage in a physical activity such as scuba diving in Hawaii, Bora Bora, or the Maldives. Perhaps you will opt to take a walking tour in Tuscany, a rafting tour in the Grand Canyon, or a kayaking adventure in Alaska. You might simply want to join a running or hiking club in your own home town. These are examples of what becomes possible when you take your life back!

Chapter THREE

A FUNDAMENTAL KNOWLEDGE OF UNHEALTHY, HIGHLY PROCESSED FOOD

This chapter will make you a food label reader for the rest of your life! You do not need to be an expert; you simply need to have a fundamental understanding of what to look for on food labels and most importantly what to avoid!

The Most Important Part of the Food Label is the Ingredient List! The healthy eating program I implemented for myself is covered in detail in Chapter 6. Before we get there, I want to identify some of the worst culprits that led to the vicious cycle surrounding my weight problem and my addiction to highly processed foods. There is no amount of exercise that will solve your weight problem on a permanent basis unless you clean up your diet. You must significantly limit your consumption of highly processed foods and focus on eating minimally processed or unprocessed foods in order to achieve permanent weight loss.

Food for Thought
- Why has the number of obese people in our society skyrocketed over the last 18 years even though we have had the luxury of a wealth of health and weight-loss information available via the Internet and other media?
- What if people were naturally inclined to consume less food and did not consider it to be deprivation?
- Why are there so many weight-loss programs that overweight people pay money for that promote eating less rather than eating right?

- Why do most dieters resume old eating patterns and regain all of their weight?

All four questions can be answered by using the following extraordinarily simple yet highly overlooked concept: *Your body must receive quality nutrients from the food you consume so that you are neither motivated to overeat nor enticed to eat the wrong foods!*

Highly Processed Food, Weight Gain, and Food Addictions

We have reached the point in this story where you can start to remove a chunk of the personal guilt and remorse that you have been heaping on yourself related to your weight problem. Put another way, your lack of will power to stop eating is mostly not your fault. Highly processed foods, even though legal and heavily promoted, contain additives that often include the following:

- Preservatives, which extend the shelf life of food.
- Flavorings, which alter the original taste of food.
- Colorings, which change the way the food looks.

You probably started eating highly processed food as a toddler. By the time you were attending all of those fun little-kid birthday parties at the fast-food restaurant du jour, you were already eating the highly processed sugar bomb euphemistically called a birthday cake. At a young age, your body was already accustomed to ingesting highly processed foods. Do you see where I am going with this?

The highly processed foods that you have consumed for years have been chemically engineered to taste good, look good, and have a long shelf life. In the process, the food is stripped of most if not all of its nutritional value. The reason that you lack will power to stop yourself from overeating at each meal and are unable to refrain from eating unhealthy snacks between meals is because your body continues to ask for the nutrients that it never receives in the highly processed foods that you constantly eat. In other words, you're eating but your body is not getting nourished. If you were consuming food that had not been so degraded through processing, your body would receive the benefits of the original nutritional value that came with that food and you would not be inclined to compulsively eat more!

A Further Understanding of Highly Processed Food

I knew on some level that eating whole, natural, healthy food must be better for me than eating food that had been highly processed. Prior to doing extensive research, I did not realize exactly how bad highly processed food was for me. Highly processed food (food that has been significantly altered from its natural state) is available and served almost everywhere that provides a venue for eating including grocery stores, fast-food establishments, restaurants, convenience stores, and gas stations with convenience stores attached. Because highly processed food is everywhere, often cheap to buy, and manufactured to look and taste appealing, we eat it and we eat it and we eat it!

One of the Worst And Most Commonly Consumed Food Groups Responsible for Weight Gain, Obesity, and Diet-Related Diseases:

Refined (Highly Processed) Carbohydrates

- Do you ever wonder why it is so easy to sit down at a restaurant and eat an entire basket of bread or biscuits before the server takes your order?
- Are you surprised that in addition to eating a salad with croutons the size of small boulders and starch-laden side dishes that accompany your entrée, you are still willing and able to tackle the dessert that appears in the middle of the table for "everyone to share"?
- Do you ever wonder why you open a box of commercially-baked cookies and none are left a half hour later?
- Are you surprised when mealtime arrives shortly after you devoured that box of cookies and you have not "spoiled your appetite"?

Welcome to the world of refined carbohydrates! When you eat refined carbs (including most breads, cereals, pastas, chips, pastries, cookies, etc.), your body receives few to no nutrients despite how much you eat. Essentially you are consuming empty calories.

Most bread is made from wheat. When wheat is refined to make white flour, most of the fiber and nutrients including the original vitamins and minerals are lost because the bran and germ have been removed from the whole grain, leaving a nutrient-poor starchy carbohydrate "bread substance." The bread is then "enriched" by adding a few synthetic vitamins and minerals. The enrichment adds minimal if any nutritional value to the bread relative to the nutrient content the wheat originally had. When you see "enriched" on a bread label, you should think "degraded food product."

Three of the Worst and Most Consumed Ingredients in Highly Processed Foods

High Fructose Corn Syrup (HFCS)

The debate rages about high fructose corn syrup. Based on my research, I am convinced that any food containing high fructose corn syrup should be avoided at all times. First of all, HFCS is a man-made sweetener designed to contain a higher amount of fructose than glucose. Similar to other man-made highly processed ingredients, HFCS enhances the taste and increases the shelf life of food. Good research clearly indicates that ingesting a significant amount of fructose interferes with your brain's ability to recognize that your body is full, which leads to the overeating we've all been doing. What a coincidence that HFCS happens to be an ingredient in just about all of the foods that we should avoid eating when we are trying to lose weight or maintain a healthy weight!

Which highly processed foods contain high fructose corn syrup? The list seems endless; however, the more common foods with HFCS are regular soft drinks, many fruit juice drinks, many commercially sold breads, sugary cereals, yogurts, cookies, cakes, crackers, jellies, jams, syrups, and soups. HFCS is often found in condiments such as barbeque sauces, ketchup, mayonnaise, and salad dressings.

HFCS exists because it is cheaper to manufacture than sucrose (table sugar). It also extends the shelf life of food and keeps it moist. High fructose corn syrup was first invented in the late 1960s and brought to market in mass production in the 1970s. The consumption of HFCS has skyrocketed since the 1970s! The number of overweight and obese people has also skyrocketed since the 1970s. Go figure!

I am convinced that HFCS has played a starring role in the increase in the number of obese people in our country over the last few decades. If you see HFCS or high fructose corn syrup on an ingredient list in a food you are about to purchase, don't buy it and definitely don't eat it!

Trans Fats
Trans fats (trans fatty acids) are terrible for you and should be avoided altogether. Specifically, I am speaking of trans fats that are created by the partial hydrogenation of oils. Trans fats alter the taste and texture, and increase the shelf life of food (a common theme for harmful ingredients found in highly processed foods). Trans fats are most commonly found in fried foods and commercially baked goods such as cookies, pies, crackers, doughnuts, and other snack foods. The consumption of trans fats, particularly in large quantities, has been shown to be a primary cause of a number of health problems—most notably coronary artery disease. When reading an ingredient list on a food label, anything that indicates that the product contains partially hydrogenated oil (i.e. partially hydrogenated vegetable oil) means that it contains trans fats and should always be avoided.

Refined Salt
Most of the salt we consume is in the highly processed foods we eat. People told me for years to lower my salt consumption, when instead they should have recommended I use a very small amount of unrefined sea salt or real salt instead of refined table salt. Additionally, they should have told me to stop eating massive quantities of highly processed foods since that is where most of our salt consumption comes from. Refined salt is found at supermarkets, restaurants, and on virtually every household dining room table and kitchen counter. Refined salt is highly processed. It has been bleached, and anti-caking agents and other harmful chemicals have been added to prevent clumping.

Even If You Already Know All This

When you read this text, do not simply shake your head if you already know these things. What you have just read is not some random theory. It relates directly to your ability to permanently lose weight.

You must reduce your consumption of refined carbohydrates as much as possible. You should also considerably limit or eliminate foods from your diet that contain high fructose corn syrup, trans fats, and refined salt in order to lose weight and keep it off permanently.

Many Restaurants Capitalize on Food-Addicted People like Crack Houses Capitalize on Drug Addicts

Think about how many times you've heard people tout a restaurant by saying "They give you really generous portions of food for what they charge." Damn right they do! The food they are serving was cheap for them to buy because it was purchased in bulk and is loaded with cheap, highly processed ingredients. My favorite examples of restaurants that serve excessive amounts of food to food-addicted people are fine steak houses, fast-food restaurants, and all-you-can-eat-buffets. I visited many fine steak houses, fast-food restaurants, and all-you-can-eat-buffets during my overweight life and I overate empty calories at each one every time.

The Steak House Dinner

Many fine or not so fine steak houses serve a basket of bread or rolls as everyone is seated at the table before any food or drinks are ordered. Once the drink orders are taken, a bottle of wine or a mixed drink in a festive glass is brought to the table and refilled throughout the meal. The basket of bread is usually refilled as the waiter or waitress takes everyone's food order or before the appetizers (which are always as large as what a normal entrée should be) arrive at the table. The salad or soup arrives soon after. The salad is loaded with cheese and boulder-size croutons, topped with a few vegetables, and drowning in a highly processed salad dressing loaded with preservatives. The soup is served in a trough and contains enough refined salt to float the

Titanic. Following the soup/salad course, the steaks from cows raised on hormones and antibiotics arrive at the table with a side of mashed potatoes, mushrooms soaking in butter, and a "healthy vegetable dish" such as asparagus which is also awash in butter (made from milk from a cow also raised on hormones and antibiotics). Once everyone's entrée is polished off, dessert appears, a dessert loaded with refined carbohydrates and highly processed sugars. It is so large it should be shared by all of the people that reside in the same zip code as the steakhouse. Amazingly, everyone at the table still has room to eat the entire thing. How is this possible? Easy! Throughout the meal, everyone at the table ingested enormous amounts of calories and barely any nutrients.

Fast-Food Restaurants

Most fast-food is easy to acquire, convenient to eat, inexpensive to buy, and usually terrible for us. There are countless menu items at fast-food restaurants that are loaded with highly processed, nutrient-poor ingredients composed of one or more of the four disastrous diet blunders: refined carbohydrates, high fructose corn syrup, trans fats, and refined salt.

People devour copious amounts of burgers, fries, fried chicken, ethnic foods, sandwiches, shakes, and desserts until they have stuffed themselves with massive portions of empty calories. Many fast-food restaurant chains entice their customers to buy large quantities of food by offering to "inexpensively" upsize the order or package multiple unhealthy items together in the same order as a "value meal."

People should never be compelled to eat more food at any restaurant because the larger size is a better value. You will learn about quick-service restaurants that actually serve high-quality, healthfully prepared food later in this book. In general, fast-food restaurants have made a significant contribution to the obesity epidemic in our society for years and should be avoided whenever possible.

All-You-Can-Eat Buffets

All-you-can-eat buffets are a highly processed food addict's nirvana. There should be a sign on the front door of the restaurant with the following truth-in-advertising slogan: "Bring your food addictions and come on in. Enjoy your weight gain. Our food is loaded with high fructose corn syrup, trans fats, refined carbohydrates, and refined salt. Please don't forget to stop by our soda fountain—it spits out chemicals like a gushing oil well. Over eat for a low price and come back tomorrow for more empty calories. We know you will be starving!"

All-you-can-eat-buffets should be avoided—always!

Highly Processed Food Is Everywhere

Think about the last time you went to a gas station that had a convenience store. Why would gas station owners want to include a convenience store as part of their business enterprise? Why wouldn't they? Similar to most establishments that serve food, gas station owners want a piece of the highly processed, food-addicted overeater market too!

Think about what's available at convenience stores: syrupy slushes, candy, chips, hot dogs, nachos, biscuits and gravy, soda pop, energy drinks, fountain drinks, cheap alcohol, simple grocery store items such as "enriched" white bread, coffee drinks served up with sugar-laden cream and artificial sweeteners, ice cream, and of course lottery tickets. The only item from the aforementioned list that doesn't harm your body is the lottery tickets! Almost all grocery stores, convenience stores, and restaurants sell food that contains highly processed ingredients.

Warehouse club retailers (i.e., Costco, Sam's Club) sell many highly processed food items in bulk and at a discount. Think about this for a minute! Consumers attempt to maximize savings by purchasing highly processed "food" in bulk as cheaply as possible and then make it their life's mission to consume everything they purchased. Who are the ultimate winners in this game?

We eat highly processed foods because they are convenient to buy and consume and made to taste good. Yet, whether you are eating highly processed foods at a restaurant, convenience store, fast food establishment, or in your own home, it is generally terrible for you. Highly processed foods contribute to poor health and obesity. In fact, I believe that the increased consumption of highly processed foods is at the root of our nationwide obesity epidemic. Although it is difficult to completely eliminate highly processed foods from our diet because such foods are present in one form or another most everywhere food is purchased, we can significantly limit our consumption of highly processed foods and eat nutrient-dense foods instead! I will show you how to successfully and conveniently accomplish this.

Chapter FOUR

A FUNDAMENTAL KNOWLEDGE OF NUTRITION

You will not succeed at weight loss by eating smaller quantities of highly processed foods that are devoid of nutrients. Permanent successful weight loss becomes possible when you eat nutrient-dense foods in moderate quantities multiple times throughout the day.

Imagine waking up each morning and knowing that the food that you are going to consume will not harm you or make you gain weight. You will easily be able to stop eating when you are full without feeling like you are depriving yourself. I wake up each morning knowing this. My diet used to be a battle of wills and now it is simple, easy, healthy, and convenient.

Consuming a diet that consists of whole, real, nutrient-rich foods will prevent you from overeating because your body will no longer crave missing nutrients.

My healthy eating program, which enabled me to lose 95 pounds in a year, consists of nutrient-dense foods. My diet is mostly comprised of lean proteins, healthy fats, and complex carbohydrates.

Important note: I did not eliminate sugar! I consume organic and raw sugar in limited quantities. Artificial sweeteners have been eliminated from my diet forever.

Carbohydrates

Attempting to significantly limit the consumption of ALL carbohydrates seems to be the Great American Weight-Loss Strategy these days as the obesity epidemic continues to spiral out of control. Fantastic, huh? Feel free to put the garbage weight-loss strategy of starving your body of carbohydrates to rest right now. Significantly limiting your carbohydrate intake could not be a more self-defeating proposition.

You must include carbohydrates in your diet because your body uses carbohydrates as its primary energy source. How are you going to function efficiently or do any meaningful exercise if you aren't consuming enough carbohydrates to provide your body with energy?

Everyone I have ever known who has attempted to severely limit carbohydrates in their diet as a weight-loss strategy (including me) has never been able to maintain it as a permanent lifestyle choice. People who choose to severely limit their carbohydrate intake might experience some initial weight loss. They will also spend a significant portion of their day feeling sluggish and enduring frequent headaches. Any exercise program they are using will ultimately cease to exist because they won't have the energy to do it.

Understanding Carbohydrates

Most carbohydrates are broken down and turned into glucose (blood sugar), which our bodies use for energy (note: fiber is a type of carbohydrate that is not converted to glucose because it cannot be digested). Carbohydrates are typically classified as simple or complex. Simple carbohydrates are composed of basic sugars and are digested (broken down) and used in the body more quickly than complex carbohydrates. Complex carbohydrates contain longer chains of sugar molecules than simple carbohydrates and provide the body with a slower and more regulated release of energy.

Rather than viewing carbohydrates from the perspective of simple carbs being bad and complex carbs being good, they should be scrutinized based on where they were sourced. Carbohydrates rich in fiber that are sourced from fruits, vegetables, whole grains, legumes, and nuts are highly beneficial and should be viewed as a crucial part of your permanent healthy eating program. Carbohydrates sourced from highly processed, nutrient-poor foods (e.g., candy, soft drinks, refined grains) should be avoided whenever possible.

Carbohydrate Planning

Generally speaking, carbohydrates should be combined with protein and consumed evenly throughout the day. The most convenient way that I have found to do this is to keep a zip lock bag of organic trail mix with me at all times. My trail mix includes almonds, walnuts, and pumpkin seeds all of which are great protein sources; as well as raisins and other dried fruits such as dried blueberries and cranberries, which are great carbohydrate sources.

The Bottom Line on Carbohydrates

Carbohydrates are the body's main source of energy and are a crucial part of a healthy diet. Anyone who recommends severely limiting or eliminating all types of carbohydrates as part of a weight-loss program is dispensing bad information because they are not advocating maintaining a healthy and sustainable lifestyle. I ate substantial amounts of highly beneficial carbohydrates in the following foods during the course of my 102-pound weight loss: Asparagus, broccoli, red onions, beans, breads made with whole grains, blueberries, raspberries, strawberries, quinoa, and sweet potatoes.

> **NOTE:** If you are experiencing a "plateau" during your weight loss and are sure that you need to lose more weight, focus on repositioning the time of day you are eating the majority of your carbohydrates. You should also increase your consumption of protein relative to the carbohydrates you are eating. You should not ever decrease your carb consumption to the point where it adversely affects your exercise or makes you walk around hungry and thinking about food all day. This is an act of deprivation and is not sustainable!

Healthy Fats

Every time I see the words "fat free" plastered across a food label (usually garbage candy sold in convenience stores and supermarkets), the first thing I remember is that food bearing this label will be very high in calories relative to nutrients and contain significant amounts of processed sugar and refined carbohydrates. I cannot imagine how many times I ate fat-free, highly processed foods during the years that I was needlessly suffering from being overweight and then obese!

During my successful weight loss, I consumed significant amounts of healthy fats—monounsaturated fats and polyunsaturated fats. I limited my consumption of saturated fats considerably and eliminated all known trans fats from my diet.

The Skinny on Fats

Monounsaturated fats and polyunsaturated fats are healthy fats that are good for us. Examples of foods that contain monounsaturated fats are avocados (which I eat most every day), olive oil (which I add to many dishes—extra virgin is the best), and nuts, such as almonds (which I eat as part of the trail mix that I consume daily). Walnuts are a great source of polyunsaturated fats. I also consume pumpkin and sunflower seeds, which contain monounsaturated and polyunsaturated fats. Various kinds of fatty fish such as trout or salmon are another way to add useful fats to your diet.

Saturated fats are mostly found in foods derived from animal products (meat, eggs, dairy). Coconut oil and palm oil also contain saturated fat. There is a lot of conflicting information about saturated fats regarding whether we should limit them in our diet or eliminate them all together. I live in the real world and believe that completely eliminating saturated fats from our diet is not realistic. I continue to significantly limit my consumption of foods that contain saturated fats on a go-forward basis just as I did over the last year during my weight loss and recommend that you do the same.

Trans fats have been discussed above, but I will reiterate my position again. Based on my research, the consumption of large amounts of trans fats has been linked to coronary artery disease, fatty liver disease, and obesity. Assuming your objective is to lose weight and live longer, eliminate trans fats from your diet.

Lean Protein

Protein is the least controversial of all the macronutrients. You must include significant amounts of protein in your diet every day. Protein in my diet comes from many different sources:

Lean chicken meat that is not processed: (healthy chicken meat comes from a chicken that was not subjected to antibiotic injections or growth hormones, and was not fed an unhealthy diet of corn and corn by-products). When you are at the grocery store, look for a healthy, cooked, organic, whole, free-range chicken.

Egg whites from organic eggs: I do not have an issue with the yolks; I simply prefer the whites. If you are trying to keep your cholesterol in check, eat only the whites.

Fish: I mostly eat tuna and halibut; however, there are many different types of healthy fish that provide an excellent source of protein including salmon, trout, and sardines. Fatty fish is a rich source of omega-3 fatty acids, which have a multitude of health attributes—most significantly they are thought to lower the risk of death from heart disease.

Beans: Beans are a great source of protein, very high in fiber, and a regular part of my diet. I highly recommend including beans in your diet. Black, kidney, pinto, navy, and lima beans are all very healthy types of beans.

Lean beef: I no longer eat beef and recommend that if you consume beef that you do so in very small quantities and choose to only eat beef from grass-fed animals not given hormones or antibiotics. Although grass-fed beef is a source of protein, it does not contain as many omega-3 fatty acids as fatty fish.

Vegetables: Vegetables are a great source of protein. Eating vegetables such as asparagus and broccoli in different dishes multiple times each week will help facilitate your protein consumption.

My specific eating program is explained in the next chapters. The purpose of this chapter is to provide a general understanding of nutrition based on my research and successful weight loss. Most importantly, the information you have just read supports the concept that your successful permanent weight loss will be predicated on your eating nutrient-dense food instead of attempting to eat smaller quantities of nutrient-poor food. Although there are many variables related to each individual person enjoying a successful permanent weight loss, consuming significant amounts of protein relative to carbohydrates, healthy fats, and sugar is extremely important and should be implemented throughout your weight-loss program.

Beginning Your Life-Changing Weight-Loss Program

My comprehensive weight-loss program is described in the next four chapters. Chapter 5 provides information and guidance on completing a cleanse. Chapter 6 offers strategies for conveniently incorporating a healthy diet into your life and gives specific ideas and examples of foods that can become a part of your permanent healthy-eating program. Chapter 7 shows you how to incorporate a meaningful exercise program into your life. Chapter 8 guides you through your first three weeks on my weight-loss program.

Specifically, I will help you accomplish your cleanse, transition into a permanent healthy-eating program, and get you on a sustainable weight-loss exercise program. When you have completed the first three weeks on my program, you will have lost a significant amount of weight, you will know that you are on the right path, and you will have mentally committed to giving yourself the huge life upgrade that you both need and deserve.

Before you get started, please remember that it is critically important for you to be willing to try new things. You must be amenable to making changes in your life so that you can live a healthy, longer life. You will be surprised by how quickly you can travel down the weight-loss path toward a healthy life if you give yourself the opportunity.

Using my weight-loss program will free you from having any desire to revert back to your previous unhealthy lifestyle! You will enjoy your new healthy-eating program immensely! You will think about food differently. You will not only enjoy the experience of eating food that contains real nutrients—you will view food from the perspective that it nourishes your body and fuels your exercise instead of viewing it as an act of deprivation or a guilty pleasure!

You do not know who you are until you have seen who you can become!

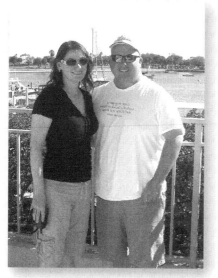

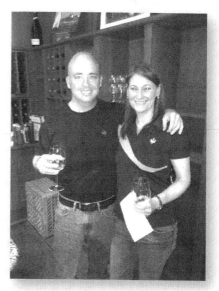

Jase and Lisa two months before Jase began his final weight loss.

Jase and Lisa at King Estate Winery toasting Jase's 102 pounds of weight loss.

Chapter FIVE

A CLEANSE TO REMOVE TOXINS AND BEGIN YOUR LIFE-CHANGING WEIGHT LOSS

Assuming you are overweight and/or clinically obese, we can immediately arrive at the conclusion that everything you have tried up until this point to lose weight and keep it off has not worked. You have a tremendous desire to free yourself from an intolerable way of living as an overweight person with food cravings and addictions. Due to your existing eating habits, you have accumulated a multitude of toxins in various parts of your body.

In order to carry out an effective weight loss, change the way you think about food, and change your life, you must rid your body of as many of these toxins as possible. The best way to accomplish all of these objectives in a short time is to use a cleanse. Completing a cleanse also resets your digestive system so that you will obtain the maximum benefit from your new healthy diet. I successfully used the Master Cleanse to jump start my life-changing weight loss. Before we get into the details of the Master Cleanse, please read the list all of the benefits that I received from doing this!

Benefits I Received during My Two Weeks on the Master Cleanse
- I developed a habit of drinking a substantial amount of water each day. This became a critical aspect of my successful weight-loss and permanent weight-maintenance program.
- I started breathing much better while I was on the cleanse.
- I stopped snoring during the third day I was on the cleanse (I used to snore and stop breathing during sleep).

- I stopped feeling aches and pains in parts of my body that were sore every day.
- I became mentally committed to the idea that I was losing weight and taking it off for the last time.
- I developed an aversion to highly processed foods, which made transitioning into a healthy eating program much easier—to this day I never feel like I am sacrificing enjoyment by eating healthy.
- I removed toxins, mucus, and plaque from my body, which allowed me to dramatically increase my energy.
- My skin cleared up.
- I experienced dramatic weight loss, which gave me the mental commitment to change my life and lose all of the remaining weight I needed to lose.

The Master Cleanse vs. Other Cleanses

Many cleanses are available for people to use to detoxify their digestive systems and eliminate toxins. I cannot comment on the effectiveness of any cleanse other than the Master Cleanse and will not speculate on how other cleanses compare. I will not limit your cleanse options to only using the Master Cleanse as the first step of my program. That said, should you decide to use another cleanse, do not eat <u>ANY</u> highly processed foods while on your chosen cleanse—you must only consume real, whole foods in their purest form (organic whenever possible). Additionally, you should choose a cleanse that is convenient to implement, includes drinking a substantial amount of water, and lasts a minimum of ten days. This could be as simple as using a raw food cleanse.

Remember, the objective of a cleanse is to rid your body of the toxins it has accumulated as a direct result of the poor diet choices that you have made. When you emerge from your chosen cleanse, you should have lost a significant amount of weight. You should also be committed to losing the rest of the weight you need to lose. You might find that you are repulsed by the food served at most restaurants, containing highly processed ingredients such as trans fats, high fructose corn syrup, refined carbohydrates, and excess sodium. You will most likely desire only wholesome, healthfully prepared food and never feel like you have to force yourself to stop eating. Most importantly, your cleanse should be a life-changing experience and you should be permanently committed to living a healthier life! Everything I just described is what the Master Cleanse did for me.

The Mental Commitment to Weight Loss through the Master Cleanse

I found the Master Cleanse to be extraordinarily beneficial in every regard. From a mental perspective, completing the Master Cleanse is the ultimate commitment to weight loss, living healthy, and changing your life. People in your life who know you are on the Master Cleanse will say things like "wow, that is hard core" and "you seem like you are serious this time." They might also say "you are out of your mind" or "you will never make it." The "you are out of your mind" and "you will never make it" comments that people said to me only strengthened my resolve to complete my two weeks on the Master Cleanse. You can use positive and negative feedback to your advantage!

In order for the Master Cleanse to be effective, you need to use it for a minimum of ten days and allow three days to gently come off of the cleanse (more on this later). I committed two weeks to the Master Cleanse and used three days to transition off. Should you decide to use the Master Cleanse, you may choose to use it for the ten-day minimum requirement or you may decide to use it for a longer period of time like I did. You will know that your cleanse has been successful if you feel better as a result of having eliminated a substantial amount of toxins from your body and changed your outlook on what your future diet will be.

IMPORTANT: The Master Cleanse is often referred to as a "diet." I would rather you view the Master Cleanse as "the first step" or "phase 1" of your life-changing weight-loss program. Remember, the primary purpose of using the Master Cleanse is to remove toxins and other impurities from your body. Removing toxins and impurities will improve the functioning of your body, which will help your weight loss be much more efficient!

Before Starting the Cleanse

You should consult with your doctor and receive medical clearance before beginning the Master Cleanse. Obviously if you have a medical condition that would make the Master Cleanse a dangerous proposition, you should not do it! Ask your doctor for an alternative cleanse recommendation if you are told that the Master Cleanse is not a viable option for you.

IMPORTANT: If your doctor questions the effectiveness of the Master Cleanse, this should not be a deterrent for you. You should seek medical clearance based on the circumstances related to your own personal medical conditions. Put another way, if your doctor says "I don't think it will work" or "performing a cleanse might be a waste of your time," you should interpret it differently than "based on your current medical condition and previous medical history, you are putting yourself at risk." If your doctor indicates that you should not use the Master Cleanse because it is medically unsafe for you, ask for an alternative recommendation.

Preparing Yourself for the Master Cleanse

Many people who have successfully used the Master Cleanse suggest consuming a vegetarian or vegan diet a few days before starting the cleanse. It has been suggested that eliminating caffeinated drinks from the diet a few days prior to starting the Master Cleanse is also a good idea. Both of these suggestions seem fantastic; however, I personally cannot speak to their effectiveness. The day I started the Master

Cleanse was the first day I began my life change—I ripped off the scab and hoped for the best. This probably made life much harder on me during the initial days I was on the cleanse; however, I successfully completed the cleanse, transitioned into a permanent healthy-eating program, and lost 95 pounds in one year (102 pounds total)!

Can Someone Really Survive and Function for Ten or More Days Without Eating Anything?

I was asked this question and many others during my two weeks on the Master Cleanse. My favorites were these two: You have not eaten anything for how many days? How are you still standing?

The truth is that I did not CHEW anything while I was on the Master Cleanse. I ingested significant amounts of vitamins, minerals, and other nutrients that I received from the maple syrup and lemons while I was on the cleanse. A few people speculated that the Master Cleanse "sounded unsafe" because they assumed that one does not ingest any protein while they are on it. This is not true. In addition to being rich in vitamins, organic lemons do contain some protein (slightly less than a gram per lemon)!

IMPORTANT: The goal of the Master Cleanse is not to consume a significant amount of protein! The goal of the Master Cleanse is to remove toxins and other impurities from your body. You are consuming plenty of vitamins, minerals, and other nutrients to sustain you while you are on the Master Cleanse. You <u>are not</u> consuming highly processed, nutrient-poor garbage that got you in trouble in the first place!

A Note to All Hard Core Master Cleanse Followers

In this chapter I describe the way I used the Master Cleanse as the first step in my life-changing weight-loss program. The ultimate goal of this book is to help as many overweight/obese people as possible commit to changing their lives using the same convenient and effective weight-loss techniques that I did. My program gives people the option of choosing an alternative cleanse so long as they consume only real, whole, foods in their most pure form while on their chosen cleanse.

I have known people who have started the Master Cleanse who were not able to meet the minimum ten-day requirement because they were unable to conveniently incorporate it into their hectic lives. Functionally speaking, the Master Cleanse could be followed most effectively by people who would have the luxury of taking time away from their personal obligations and work schedules to focus exclusively on following the precise steps of the program as it was originally designed by Stanley Burroughs in the 1940s. This sounds great but it is unrealistic.

I implemented incidental modifications as a matter of convenience and necessity during my two weeks on the Master Cleanse. These incidental modifications did not have an adverse effect on the success of my weight loss or my dedication to a healthier way of eating and thinking about food. Additionally, I am certain that I was able to eliminate most of the toxins and impurities in my own body throughout the two-week period that I was on the Master Cleanse. Although I may not have performed the Master Cleanse exactly as a purist would recommend, my life-changing weight-loss and weight-maintenance results have been fantastic.

Preparing the Master Cleanse Mixture

You should consume eight or more 10-oz. servings each day of the Master Cleanse drink prepared using the following ingredients:

- Lemon juice squeezed from organic lemons
- Organic Grade B dark amber maple syrup
- Cayenne pepper (tincture form)
- Purified water

IMPORTANT:

- Organic lemons means organic lemons!
- Organic Grade B dark amber maple syrup means organic Grade B dark amber maple syrup!

You must start viewing nutrition differently right now! Lemon juice from concentrate and refined highly processed maple syrup that has been stripped of essential nutrients and loaded with extra sugar and chemicals can <u>NOT</u> be used as a substitute for organic lemons and organic Grade B dark amber maple syrup. Your new healthy lifestyle starts now! The organic lemons and organic Grade B dark amber maple syrup contain the proper nutrients to see you through the Master Cleanse.

One 10-oz. Serving of the Master Cleanse Recipe

- 2 tablespoons (one ounce) of lemon juice (the juice from about ½ lemon)
- 2 tablespoons (one ounce) of organic Grade B dark amber maple syrup
- 8 ounces of filtered water (no flavored water or water with additives)
- 2 drops of cayenne tincture (individual drops, not dropper-fulls)

Making the Master Cleanse Convenient

Ideally, you would take a vacation from work and personal obligations and focus only on the Master Cleanse. The mixture would be prepared and consumed as individually prepared servings eight or more times each day. This is unrealistic for nearly everyone. I am going to assume that you have a busy schedule and are constantly fighting the clock and meeting deadlines, or that you might have to travel as a part of your work schedule like I do.

I recommend making enough Master Cleanse mixture each morning to last the entire day. In order to do this, fill a one-gallon container with enough mixture to provide eight (8) 10-oz. individual servings for the day. Only the cayenne tincture should be added with each individual serving just before consuming.

IMPORTANT: You may consume as much of the Master Cleanse Mixture as you wish each day—you are not limited to 80 ounces.

Preparing a Daily Quantity of Servings

1. Squeeze enough organic lemons to create one cup of organic lemon juice. Pour into a one gallon container (a funnel really helps!)
2. Add one cup of Grade B dark amber maple syrup.
3. Add eight cups (a half gallon) of purified water to the mixture. The result is 80 ounces or 8 10-oz. servings.
4. Do not pre-mix the cayenne—it should not steep in the mixture.

Your gallon jug holding the Master Cleanse mixture, a 10-oz. mug, and bottle of cayenne tincture should be with you constantly while you are on the cleanse. Always stir or shake the mixture before pouring an individual serving. When you have poured an individual serving into your container, add 2 single drops of cayenne tincture, stir again, and consume. Should you prefer the mixture warm or hot (I did), heat in a microwave or on a stove before adding the cayenne tincture.

Assisting Your Body with Eliminating Toxins And Impurities

You will need to help the effectiveness of the Master Cleanse by promoting the elimination of toxins. In other words, you don't want to release the toxins inside your body without completely eliminating them from your body. You accomplish this by drinking lots of water and using a mild laxative during the cleanse. For the laxative effect, you can take an herbal laxative, drink a laxative tea, or use an internal salt water bath. I never ingested an herbal laxative and did not use an internal salt water bath so I cannot comment on the effectiveness of either method. I chose to consume single servings of Organic Traditional Medicinals Smooth Move tea throughout the two weeks that I was on the Master Cleanse. I recommend consuming a single serving of an organic laxative tea starting on the first evening, then every other evening thereafter while you are on your cleanse.

While You Are on Your Cleanse, Drink Substantial Amounts of Water Every Day and Continue the Routine for the Rest of Your Life!

Drinking a plentiful amount of water each day will give you the opportunity to enjoy a successful Master Cleanse experience. You need to make this a habit for the rest of your life—it will be critically important to your current weight loss and future weight maintenance!

Before starting my weight-loss program, I not only did not drink <u>enough</u> water every day; I hardly drank any water at all. As I said before, there were many times during my overweight/obese life that the only water I consumed was the melted ice in the soft drinks or cocktails I drank. My lack of water consumption was terrible for me and played a significant role in my being so overweight.

Many variables determine the appropriate amount of water you should consume including the climate you live in, the amount of exercise that you engage in, and the amount of water-rich foods (mostly found in fruits and vegetables) you eat on a regular basis. I drink a minimum of three-quarters of a gallon of water every day—most days I drink a gallon of water. One easy rule of thumb you can use to determine how much water you should drink every day is this:

Divide your weight in <u>pounds</u> in half. Half of your weight in pounds equals the minimum number of <u>ounces</u> of water you should consume each day (if the amount based on this calculation is greater than a gallon, drink at least a gallon of water each day and continue to drink whatever amount is comfortable beyond that). Example: A 200-pound person should consume no less than 100 ounces of water each day.

What to Expect During the Cleanse

Everyone will have their own unique experiences on the Master Cleanse. Some might experience headaches and/or body aches while others will not. The reason you might experience head or body aches is because your body is detoxifying. Feeling discomfort during detoxification is not unusual. Although it is not recommended in any book I have read describing how to use the Master Cleanse, I decided to take a couple of Advil (my personal choice) immediately when I experienced discomfort.

I know this is frowned upon by many who have deep convictions regarding how the Master Cleanse should be performed; however, I refused to try to function in pain. In addition to other over-the-counter pain medications, there are natural herbal remedies you might want to consider if you experience discomfort during your cleanse.

It is important to remember that a major role of the water you are consuming during the cleanse is to eliminate toxins from your body. Consuming the appropriate amount of water will help to eliminate or decrease the severity of potential discomforts while you are on your cleanse.

Emerging from the Master Cleanse

Once you have completed the Master Cleanse, you <u>MUST</u> come off of it easily and gently! Remember, you will have not eaten solid food for at least 10 days (in my case, 14 days). You do not want to cause undue stress on your digestive system.

- During the first day you should consume only fresh squeezed organic orange juice (pineapple juice is an acceptable substitution). Drink the juice slowly and try to consume five or six 8-oz. glasses throughout the day.

- During the second day, incorporate some organic low or no sodium soup or vegetable broth into your diet. Try to consume five or six small servings throughout the day.

- The third day, eat five or six small servings of organic fruits and vegetables. Be sure to chew each bite thoroughly.

- The fourth day, you are free to begin your permanent healthy-eating program (described in the next chapter).

When you complete your cleanse, you will find yourself eating a minimum of five or six small portions of food throughout the day. Eating small-portion meals and snacks throughout the day will help regulate your blood sugar and reduce the total amount of food you will eat. Eating small-portion foods coupled with drinking water early and often throughout the day is absolutely essential for permanent and substantial weight loss.

Comprehending What You Have Just Accomplished
Once you have completed ten or more days on the Master Cleanse, you should be very proud of what you have just accomplished! Although highly rewarding, it is not easy and proves that you are committed to your health. You will be feeling, breathing, and sleeping better. You will have lost a substantial amount of weight in a short time, ridding your body of harmful and unnecessary toxins. You will have also prepared your body and mind to efficiently lose the rest of the weight you need to lose. You should have no doubt that you will be extraordinarily successful losing all of your remaining weight.

Start to dream big—imagine how much better your life is going to be when you have taken the remainder of your weight off once and for all! Turn the page and discover all of the incredible food options that are available for you to enjoy as part of your lifelong healthy eating program. Know that the transition will be so much easier now that you have detoxified your body. Your mental commitment to a permanent healthy eating program should be easy now that you have completed the Master Cleanse.

Chapter SIX

ESTABLISHING A PERMANENT HEALTHY EATING PROGRAM

Your attitude and approach to food should be as follows: Food provides my body with nutrients, fuels my exercise, and should always be enjoyed.

The most important concept of the healthy eating program: Approximately 75% of your current weight-loss and future weight-maintenance success will depend on consuming a proper diet!

Given the importance of diet as it relates to successful weight loss, you should ask yourself the following question every time you eat:

What is the nutrient content of what I am about to put in my mouth?

Are you receiving actual nutrients from what you are eating or are you about to consume highly processed food that will provide your body with little or no nutrition?

The balance of macronutrients (carbs, fats, and proteins) consumed during weight loss is important; however, your primary concern should always be analyzing the ingredient list associated with the food you are eating. The easiest rule to follow is the more highly processed the food, the worse it is for you. Your body has little to no use for highly processed food and does not use it efficiently!

After determining that your food choice has solid nutrient content (meaning that it is minimally processed or unprocessed), you should focus on your macronutrient ratios. Consuming significant amounts of protein balanced with complex carbohydrates, healthy fats, and limited amounts of organic raw or natural sugar is highly beneficial for weight loss. My permanent healthy-eating program offers many food options and a variety of methods that make healthy eating convenient. Convenience is the key critical component to any weight-loss and weight-maintenance program. In order to conveniently eat healthy, you must strategize your new diet.

Strategizing a New Diet

Having read the first five chapters of this book, you are more than aware that the primary objective of proper diet is to significantly limit your consumption of highly processed foods (which are mostly devoid of nutrients) and eat nutrient-dense foods instead. Many overweight people consider healthy eating to be impossible because they think they don't have time. I will help you overcome this false perception. Use the information provided in this chapter to strategize how you are going to accommodate eating healthy into your life.

We humans are creatures of habit. We go to the same grocery stores and replace food items we use in our kitchens. We know exactly where to find these items in the grocery store because we have replaced them so many times.

When we purchase meals from restaurants, we purchase the same meals from familiar restaurants repeatedly. When a new restaurant is added to the mix, we memorize their menu and the same meals become regular selections from the new restaurant.

You have read many times that in order to lose weight and keep it off permanently, you must make a lifestyle change. Strategizing a new diet is an important part of the lifestyle change that you will make in order to lose weight and keep it off permanently.

Removing Limitations: Tips for Making Your New Healthy Eating Program Flexible and Efficient

Important Factors to Consider When Analyzing Food Costs

You will spend more money when you buy healthy, unprocessed food instead of highly processed pretend food. You pay more for labels that read **ORGANIC, REAL,** and **ALL NATURAL** instead of labels that have an ingredient list with words you can't pronounce running down the entire length of the packaging. Although you will spend a little more money to eat healthy, it is important to remember the following:

- When you consume minimally processed or unprocessed food, you eat less because your body is actually receiving the nutrients that it needs from the food you are eating.
- You will buy smaller quantities of food because you are naturally inclined to eat less.
- The extra money you spend on healthy (minimally processed or unprocessed) food will pay for itself many times over given what you will save on current and future healthcare expenses.
- The money you spend on healthy food will also pay for itself many times over because you will feel great, you will have an increased enjoyment of life, and you will be more productive in all areas of your life.

Controlling Portion Sizes

As soon as your body is accustomed to receiving substantial nutrients from the small meals you are eating, you will find that you no longer need to be as focused on portion control. If you continue to feel challenged by portion control once you are consistently eating nutrient-dense foods, you are most likely not following another aspect of my program (i.e. drinking enough water).

When you start your new healthy eating program, you need to think about portion control in terms of defining a "small" meal. A great way to start portion control is to downsize the plates and bowls you use. Instead of using plates that are 12 inches (or larger) in diameter, use plates that are approximately 8 inches (or smaller) in diameter. Instead of using bowls that can hold three or more cups of water, use bowls that hold no more than one cup of water. You can select bowls yourself by filling a measuring cup with water and pouring the water into different size bowls.

Organic Food

There are differing opinions regarding whether it is worth it to buy organic food. By consuming organic foods, you limit your exposure to pesticides including the insecticides, fungicides, and herbicides found in many fruits and vegetables. You also limit your consumption of hormones and antibiotics found in meat and dairy products. Organic foods are not genetically modified or irradiated.

Food manufacturers are required to go through third-party certification standards and be in compliance with USDA organic regulations in order to be able to place the USDA ORGANIC seal on their food packaging. Products labeled "100% Organic" must contain 100% organic ingredients. Products labeled "Organic" must contain a minimum of 95% organic ingredients, and the other 5% must comply with other restrictions such as no genetically modified organisms (GMOs). If a food product is labeled "Made with Organic Ingredients," it must contain a minimum of 70% organic ingredients and the other 30% must comply with other restrictions and include no GMOs. Products that contain less than 70% organic ingredients may list the organic ingredients on the side of the packaging but may not make any organic claim on the front of the package.

Bottom line, organic food is usually more expensive. That said, choosing to buy and eat organic food whenever possible signifies that you are making an investment in the health and well-being of yourself and your family. In the grand scheme of things, is there a better financial investment?

Further Confirmation of Why it is Important to Limit Highly processed Foods in Your Diet

Many chemicals contained in highly processed foods are not recognized by the body. The body does not have any use for these substances and treats them as if they are foreign and possibly toxic. Toxic substances are stored in fat cells in the body. The most important reason I recommend starting my weight-loss program with a cleanse is to enable your body to eliminate toxins. The reason I recommend drinking a substantial amount of water every day is because water facilitates the elimination of toxins being released from your fat cells.

Making a List of Easy-to-Prepare and -Assemble Foods

My own list of easy-to-prepare and easy-to-assemble food options are provided in this book. You should make a list of ten or more healthy food items that you can prepare in a very short amount of time—ideally seven minutes or less. Of your ten food items, five should be available to you at your home or work place at all times. Feel free to use any or all of the choices on my example list to supplement your own list. The most important idea when creating your list is that your food choices must contain minimal or no highly processed ingredients.

Earlier I described how I used to eat when I was overweight—I would either start my day with an unhealthy breakfast and eat poorly throughout the day or let a significant portion of the day lapse without eating anything. Eventually I would be starving and eat whatever food was most readily available regardless of how bad it was for me. Having healthy meals available that can be prepared or assembled in seven minutes or less solved that problem once and for all.

Eating Family Meals at Home

The Challenge: Satisfying Everyone's Preferences

You arrive home from work and either you or your spouse has to prepare dinner for the family. If you have children, dinner has to feed multiple people. With work and school schedules, family dinners are the only time during the week that everyone has a chance to spend time together. You and your spouse do not have time to prepare different meals to accommodate everyone's preferences and diet restrictions.

The Solution

You have chosen to live a healthy lifestyle. You should have meal options that you can prepare for yourself in seven minutes or less while preparing food for everyone else. I provide examples in this chapter of how to do this. You do not have to give up your weight-loss commitment and eat the same food everyone is eating in order to spend time with your family during meals. You can enjoy each other's company and not eat the same food. Other members of your family might wish to join you in your healthy eating program. Imagine how great it would be if your children were inclined to eat healthy starting at an early age!

Restaurant Choices

The Challenge: Choosing Restaurants That Prepare and Serve Tasty, Healthfully Prepared Food

Although eating out is generally the more expensive option, people choose to dine out at restaurants frequently because of time constraints associated with work and personal obligations. Meetings and social events are conducted over meals. Most restaurants make money by purchasing highly processed food in bulk as cheaply as possible. The highly processed food is prepared and served for the most money restaurants can charge while convincing the patrons they received a great deal on their meal. The result is the patrons eat nutrient-poor, highly processed foods that have been chemically altered to taste great. They are unaware of what the true taste of the food they are eating should be because their taste buds have been desensitized for years from eating highly processed junk.

The Solution:

Most cities have one or more restaurants that serve food prepared with healthy, minimally processed or unprocessed ingredients (see below for some examples I've found). Having healthfully prepared, minimally processed or unprocessed food purchased from restaurants readily available in your home or work place means that you have added to your list of available foods that can be assembled in seven minutes or less!

IMPORTANT: Do not assume restaurants that serve healthfully prepared foods are the most expensive! The restaurants listed on the following pages are moderately priced and less expensive than many restaurants that serve highly processed food. Some of the nicest and most expensive restaurants I frequented during my overweight/obese years served highly processed garbage that was beautifully described on the menu! Highly processed foods are not exclusively found at fast-food establishments, gas stations, and convenience stores!

Instead of eating at restaurants that mostly offer highly processed food on their menus, start frequenting restaurants in your community that serve nutritious, wholesome food and support your local economy. Eugene and many other cities are privileged to have restaurants such as these. When you make a conscious decision to eat at restaurants that mostly offer wholesome food that is either unprocessed or minimally processed (where most or all of the nutrients are still present), you are making a choice that is consistent with someone who wants to lose weight and keep it off permanently. Become familiar with the menu at these establishments and incorporate healthy, minimally processed and unprocessed foods into your permanent healthy-eating program! Do not ever presume that restaurants that serve healthy foods are only the expensive restaurants!

Creswell Coffee Co. (the place where I first discussed my life-changing weight-loss goals with my wife, Lisa) is a restaurant located in the very small town where I live, Creswell, Oregon, which has a population of just over 5,000 people. Creswell Coffee Co. serves organic fair-trade coffee, homemade soups, and salads using locally grown produce. You can learn more about Creswell Coffee at www.creswellcoffeeco.com. If you live in a small community, you should be able to find local coffee shops or cafes that offer nutritious, healthfully prepared foods also!

> **IMPORTANT:** Prior to selecting restaurants that you want to include as part of your new healthy eating program, find out how their food is prepared.

The Green Salmon Coffee and Tea House (www.thegreensalmon. com), one of my favorite small town restaurants in the world, is located in the tiny coastal town of Yachats, Oregon. The Green Salmon Coffee and Tea House offers an organic menu of scones, croissants, salads, and panini sandwiches. The coffee drinks are made using the highest quality and most flavorful organic fair-trade beans. They also serve a variety of organic hot chocolates, organic smoothies, and exceptional teas from around the world.

> **IMPORTANT:** When you travel out of town for pleasure or work and you find yourself in a small town, ask the locals what their favorite restaurants or cafes are that serve healthfully prepared food.

Café Yumm (www.cafeyumm.com) is another one of my favorite restaurants. They currently have locations in several cities in Oregon. Café Yumm offers a great selection of healthy, nutritious entrées, sauces, and dressings that I eat with other foods on my Healthy and Convenient Food List (provided in a few pages). The items that I most frequently purchase are Yumm Bowls and Roasted Garlic Yumm Sauce. Yumm Bowls are delicious and conveniently offered in small, medium, and large sizes and can be customized in many different ways. All ingredients in Yumm Bowls can be easily substituted to accommodate nutrition and diet preferences. I typically order two large Yumm Bowls (with extra avocado) and divide them into four different meals over two days. We always keep Roasted Garlic Yumm Sauce in our refrigerator and enjoy it with salads, sandwiches, vegetables, hard-boiled eggs, and other dishes.

Chipotle Mexican Grill (www.chipotle.com) is an example of a large successful chain restaurant that offers healthier menu options than most. We are fortunate to have one in Eugene. I eat healthy, convenient food at home from Chipotle Mexican Grill on a regular basis. I bring home sides of grilled fajita chicken and cooked vegetables and store them in my refrigerator. I include their chicken and vegetables in different stir-fries and other meals that are prepared and assembled in seven minutes or less.

Summary on Dining Out

Whenever possible, you should only frequent restaurants that offer wholesome, unprocessed or minimally processed foods on their menu. If you dine out on a regular basis, you should identify restaurants in or near your own town that offer nutritious-items on their menu. Eating healthy meals from restaurants that you visit on a regular basis will add another aspect of convenience to your permanent healthy-eating program.

You will be forced to eat at restaurants sometimes that mostly offer highly processed foods on their menu (remember, these restaurants can range from being inexpensive to very expensive). You won't get to pick the restaurant if you are attending someone else's birthday party. You won't get to pick the restaurant if you are attending a business meeting hosted by someone else. You probably won't get to pick the restaurant very often if you frequently dine with your boss during your work day. The best advice for these occasions is to turn a negative into a positive and order the baked or grilled fish option on the menu. You may not know the source of the fish, but, on average, it usually is the much healthier choice found on an unhealthy menu. A healthy salad with dressing on the side that is unprocessed or minimally processed is another good choice.

Buying Prepared Food for Convenience

In order to always have healthy food accessible in my kitchen, I take home high-quality prepared food from grocery stores (more on this in a minute). I am not referring to boxed, highly processed food with an ingredient list a mile long. I am referring to food that is prepared using whole, natural, unprocessed ingredients. The best grocery store chain I know is Whole Foods Market. If you live in a city that has a Whole Foods Market, you win! Whole Foods Market is the largest retailer of natural and organic foods. Unfortunately, there is not a Whole Foods Market in Eugene, but Eugene has Market of Choice grocery stores that offer a large variety of high-quality foods including foods prepared in their own store kitchen. You should consistently use the grocery store in your area that offers the greatest selection of healthy foods.

> **Note:** You can minimize the time you spend buying food if you are able to conveniently buy healthy foods at restaurants and grocery stores that are near each other in the same shopping trip. Convenience is extremely important when you are incorporating healthy eating into your life!

Preparing Your Own Convenience Food

Buying prepared food is usually more expensive than buying individual ingredients and preparing food yourself. Whether you are buying prepared food or preparing food yourself, keep sealable storage containers in your kitchen at all times. Sealable storage containers will enable you to easily access chopped vegetables, individual servings of fruit, cooked meat and poultry, and prepared meals from your refrigerator. Sealable storage containers are also convenient for transporting individual servings of food to your place of work—remember, you must be able to conveniently prepare and assemble healthy meals in seven minutes or less!

If you are preparing your own food—including chopping your own vegetables, cooking, and separating individual servings, block out a specific period of time (usually no more than an hour) twice during each week and prepare everything at once. Since you will be eating multiple times each day, you do not want to be preparing and cooking each individual meal.

Healthy and Convenient Food List

Healthy Convenient Foods Purchased From a Grocery Store

Organic Trail Mix

Health:

My organic trail mix contains organic dried cranberries, organic raw sunflower seeds, organic whole raw almonds, organic raw cashews, organic raw pumpkin seeds, organic raisins, and organic walnuts. It's a great source of protein, carbs, and healthy fat.

Convenience:

Although there are unlimited options available to you as part of your new healthy-eating program, I highly recommend incorporating organic trail mix into your diet. Organic trail mix should be purchased in bulk and should always be available to you whether you are at your home, at your workplace, or traveling. Most good supermarkets carry several organic trail mixes with a variety of healthy ingredients that will satisfy nearly everyone's palate. Organic trail mix is the most convenient source of nutrition on my list. I eat organic trail mix by itself as a snack, mix it into my yogurt in the morning for breakfast, mix it into my salad at lunch, and use it as a side dish with meals. Preparation and assembly time—none!

> **Note:** If you choose to buy pre-packaged trail mix instead of buying it in bulk, read the label! Many pre-packaged trail mixes contain refined sugars, salts or other processed flavor enhancers.

Yogurt

FAGE All Natural Low-Fat (2%) Greek Strained Yogurt

Health:

High-protein yogurt is a great option for people who are not lactose-intolerant. FAGE uses all natural ingredients. I eat this particular brand of yogurt because it is protein-rich, gluten-free, and contains no added sweeteners or preservatives. I mainly eat yogurt for breakfast and use approximately 3/4 of a cup of 2% plain yogurt and add in organic trail mix, organic muesli (purchased in bulk), and 1.5 tablespoons of organic Grade B maple syrup and a little organic sugar.

Convenience:

I purchase two 35.3-oz. tubs of yogurt at the grocery store. We eat a lot of Greek yogurt and use it with a variety of easy-to-assemble and -prepare foods. The preparation and assembly time for my yogurt, trail mix, muesli breakfast is less than two minutes.

Organic Hard-Boiled Eggs

Health:

The diet of the laying hens greatly affects the nutritional quality of the eggs. I eat eggs that come from organic hens that are fed a 100% organic vegetarian diet. Eggs are nutrient-dense and a great source of protein. Most of the cholesterol is found in the yolk, so if you have a cholesterol problem, you can still get protein from just the egg whites. Otherwise, enjoy the yolk because it contains a lot of nutrients.

Convenience:

A good way to hard boil eggs is to use a push-pin or thumb-tack and poke a tiny hole in the fat end of the egg. Place the eggs in a pan of cold water enough to cover the eggs. Bring the water to a rapid boil. When the water starts to boil, immediately turn off the heat and cover with a lid for eight minutes. Run cold water over the eggs or place them in a bowl of cold water. Remove the egg shells as soon as the eggs have cooled. Once the shells have been removed, the eggs can be eaten immediately or stored in a sealed container in your refrigerator.

Mari's Muffins

Health:

Mari is a registered dietician who combined her love of baking and knowledge of nutrition to create a protein-packed, high-fiber meal, all in a single muffin. One of Mari's Muffins has the equivalent calories, protein, calcium, and fiber of a full breakfast consisting of (1) slice of whole wheat bread, (1/2) cup of milk, (1) serving of fruit, and (1) egg. Mari's Muffins taste great and provide a nutritious meal in a single muffin.

Convenience:

Mari's Muffins can be ordered online at **www.marismuffins.com**. Mari's muffins can be stored in the refrigerator and warmed in the microwave for thirty seconds or stored in the freezer and warmed in the microwave for one minute.

Healthy Shake

Health:

Healthy shakes are only truly healthy if they are made with high-quality ingredients. I use Dream Protein which is a hormone free whey protein. Dream Protein contains no aspartame, artificial sweeteners, added sugar, casein, or artificial ingredients. The shake by itself is a great source of protein. Mix in a handful of frozen organic blueberries and raspberries and your shake becomes a rich source of protein that is also high in fiber, antioxidants, and phytochemicals.

Convenience:

Mix one scoop of Dream Protein Powder with a hand full of frozen organic blueberries and raspberries, six ounces of distilled water or organic 2% milk, and a few ice cubes. Blend and pour. The preparation and assembly time is less than five minutes.

I order Dream Protein Powder online at Amazon.com.

IMPORTANT: Many people are involved in weight-loss programs where they are encouraged to regularly drink shakes instead of eating food as a meal. Replacing meals with shakes on a frequent basis deprives the body of whole-food sourced nutrition. To combat feeling hungry which is an inevitable result of the body being deprived of nutrients, many popular diet shakes include ingredients designed to trick the body into feeling full (resulting in another side effect which is feeling bloated).

You may include a healthy shake as one of your five or six small meals if it does not contain a bunch of harmful ingredients. Your healthy shake should always be consumed in balance with the other nutrition you are eating during the day.

Quinoa Salad:

Health:

Quinoa is gluten-free, cholesterol-free, and contains all nine essential amino acids, making it a complete protein. There are a many different ingredients that can go into making a great quinoa salad. I eat quinoa salad prepared with chopped red onions, black olives, cilantro, green peppers, tomatoes, olive oil, black beans, and almonds and try to ensure that all ingredients are organic whenever possible.

Convenience:

Quinoa Salad can usually be purchased at a restaurant, grocery store, or easily prepared in your kitchen. I have found that a pound of Quinoa Salad will last two people two days eaten in small portions with three or four meals. The preparation and assembly time for prepared Quinoa Salad is less than a minute—remove Quinoa Salad from the refrigerator and dish. Preparing your own Quinoa Salad can be part of your twice-weekly healthy food preparation.

Sonoma Chicken Salad

Health:

Chicken is a great protein source. I eat chicken that comes from barn-roaming chickens that were not raised with antibiotics, added hormones, or preservatives—instead they were raised on a 100% vegetarian diet and did not consume any animal fats or by-products. Sonoma Chicken Salad should be prepared using healthy, all natural ingredients such as Sonoma dressing made with organic canola mayonnaise and oil. Other ingredients may include sea salt, pepper, healthy nuts, and red grapes.

Convenience:

Sonoma Chicken Salad can usually be purchased at a restaurant, grocery store, or prepared in your kitchen. One pound of Sonoma Chicken Salad lasts two to three days and is portioned and consumed as three meals. Similar to other pre-made salads, preparation and assembly time is less than a minute as you just remove the Sonoma Chicken Salad from the refrigerator and dish. I eat my Sonoma Chicken Salad with organic blue corn chips and chopped lettuce.

Tuna Salad

Health:

Tuna is an excellent source of protein and there are endless tuna salad recipes. I usually eat tuna salad made with organic canola mayonnaise, green onions, diced celery, lemon juice, and sea salt.

Convenience:

Tuna salad can usually be purchased in the grocery store or prepared in your kitchen. One pound of tuna salad lasts two to three days and is portioned and consumed as three meals. Remove the tuna salad from the refrigerator and dish. Organic blue corn chips, chopped lettuce, and diced red onions make a great addition to tuna salad.

Broccoli Burst Salad

Health:

Broccoli is an excellent source of protein. I discovered Broccoli Burst Salads immediately after I completed the Master Cleanse. I could not believe how much I liked this salad the first time I tried it. The ingredients in the Broccoli Burst Salad I eat include broccoli, raisins, sunflower seeds, diced red onions, and organic canola mayonnaise dressing. Some prepared broccoli burst salads contain bacon. When bacon is present, I eat everything but the bacon.

Convenience:

Broccoli Burst Salad can be purchased at a restaurant, grocery store, or prepared in your kitchen. One pound of Broccoli Burst Salad lasts two to three days and is portioned and consumed as three or four meals. The preparation and assembly time is less than a minute—remove the Broccoli Burst Salad from the refrigerator and dish.

Avocados And Jase-Style Guacamole

Health:

It might surprise you to learn that an avocado is technically a fruit. Anyone who knows me knows that I am passionate about avocados because they are loaded with healthy nutrients. Avocados are a great source of fiber and potassium (an avocado contains more potassium than a banana). The only knock I ever hear on avocados is they are high in fat. Avocados are high in UNSATURATED FATS, which are good for your heart. I consumed many avocados throughout the course of my weight loss and continue to eat them most every day.

Convenience:

Avocados can be eaten by themselves, mixed into salads, and used to make guacamole. The healthy guacamole I prepare a few times a week consists of one organic Haas avocado, a handful of pre-chopped and bagged organic red onions, organic olive oil, organic sea salt, and organic blue corn chips (tomatoes and organic salsa may also be added to enhance the taste).

The preparation and assembly time is less than three minutes if chopped red onions are already in a sealable storage bag in the refrigerator; otherwise it may take four minutes. Peel and chop an avocado, sprinkle chopped red onions over the top of the avocado, drizzle organic olive oil over the top of the red onions, lightly salt with organic sea salt, add organic chopped tomato if you wish, and eat with a small bowl of organic blue corn chips. Holy Guacamole!

Turkey Sandwich

Health:

Turkey is an excellent source of protein. Similar to other foods on my list, a turkey sandwich is only healthy if the sandwich is prepared using the right ingredients. A turkey sandwich made with highly processed turkey meat, refined bread, unhealthy mayonnaise, served with highly processed potato chips that are high in fat and sodium is terrible for you. Alternatively, a turkey sandwich made using whole grain (100% whole grain) bread, organic mayonnaise made with cage-free eggs, organic roasted turkey breast, organic basil, and organic red onions, served with organic blue corn tortilla chips, is a much healthier option.

Convenience:

I purchase all ingredients for my turkey sandwich at the grocery store. They include sliced turkey from Applegate Organics, Dave's Killer Bread (whole grain), Spectrum Organic Mayonnaise, and organic red onion from the produce section. I eat my sandwich with simply sprouted Way Better Snacks tortilla chips. You will find the same or similar suppliers of healthy organic foods in a quality grocery store in your community.

Cooked Chicken

Health:

Chicken (skin excluded) contains more healthy fat than red meat and is an excellent source of protein. As described earlier, the type of chicken you purchase will determine how healthy it is for you. I purchase all natural or organic whole cooked chickens.

Convenience:

I purchase one whole cooked chicken at a time. When I return from the grocery store, I pull the cooked whole chicken out of the bag, remove the skin and bones, and slice the meat into pieces. I place the chicken pieces in a sealable storage container and refrigerate the sliced chicken until use. I eat chicken by itself, in salads, sandwiches, and with grilled vegetables as a full meal.

Grilled Vegetables

Health:

Grilled vegetables are a great source of nutrition and many contain significant amounts of protein, healthy carbs, and healthy fat. Grilled vegetables are always readily available in my refrigerator.

Convenience:

The easiest way to have grilled vegetables available is to purchase them (already grilled) at a grocery store or restaurant—first making sure they were grilled using a healthy marinade. Grilled organic vegetables can be obtained from most grocery stores and food coops. You should find the stores in your community that have the best combination of freshness and cost. Store grilled vegetables in an airtight container in the refrigerator and they will stay good for at least two days. My personal preference is to block out time once a week and grill vegetables during a one-hour food preparation session. I regularly eat organic grilled asparagus, zucchini, bell peppers, mushrooms, and broccoli. Other great options that you might consider include organic kale, cauliflower, chard, green beans, carrots, and red onions.

When you grill your own vegetables, use very little marinade (this prevents them from becoming soggy) and always store in an air-tight container in the refrigerator. Grilled vegetables can be reheated using a healthy marinade (i.e., a little organic olive oil and sprinkled organic sea salt) at mealtime. Marinades can be used as dipping sauces. I purchase all of my healthy marinades other than organic olive oil combined with organic sea salt at a very reasonable price from local restaurants and store them in my refrigerator. Preparation and assembly time for prepared grilled vegetables stored in the refrigerator is less than two minutes.

Frozen Foods

Health:

There are many healthy unprocessed frozen foods options available at quality grocery stores. Keeping convenient, healthy frozen food in the freezer is a great idea as family and friends can drop in unexpectedly at mealtime. Do not stock large boxes of processed foods in the freezer. Instead of being the family that dumps frozen corn dogs covered with ice crystals on a heating pan when your children's friends arrive at your house at mealtime, be the family that efficiently prepares a healthy stir fry using an organic vegetable medley of green beans, broccoli, carrots, red peppers, onions, and mushrooms, mixed with organic or all natural chicken.

Convenience:

I buy boxes of Cascadian Farms organic frozen vegetables from the grocery store and keep them in our freezer. In order to prepare and enjoy a quick meal, I remove the vegetables from the packaging and heat with some pre-cooked chicken (found in an airtight storage container in our refrigerator). This meal can either be heated in a large bowl in the microwave or in a large stir-fry pan on the stove. To save time, I thaw the vegetables in the microwave, mix in a healthy marinade, and finish cooking in a pan on the stove. Because the packaged vegetables are already chopped, preparation and assembly takes no more than seven minutes.

Healthy Convenient Foods Purchased from Restaurants

Below is a list of convenience foods I purchase from restaurants in my community to provide examples of take-out foods that you should consider when you purchase healthfully prepared foods from restaurants in your own community. Remember that the cost of eating food from a healthy, moderately priced menu will not be as expensive as you think. You will eat less food because healthier food is more nutrient-dense, and you will require fewer calories to feel satiated as you continue to lose weight.

Restaurant: Creswell Coffee Co.
Restaurant Type: Coffee Shop/Café
Prepared Foods I Take Home: Minty Snap Pea Salad, Quinoa Salad, and Broccoli Burst Salad
Health and Convenience: Creswell Coffee Co. offers a variety of healthy food including great salads, which can be enjoyed at their coffee shop or taken to go. Minty Snap Pea Salad, Quinoa Salad, and Broccoli Burst Salads are my favorites. If I have time, I eat a part of a large salad in the restaurant (sometimes for breakfast in the morning— more on this later), and take home the rest in a "to go" container to be enjoyed as another meal.

Restaurant: Café Yumm
Restaurant Type: Casual Dining
Prepared Foods I Take Home: Original Yumm Bowl with extra avocado, Chilean Zucchini Bowl, Roasted Garlic Yumm Sauce, Jalapeno Sesame Salsa
Health and Convenience: The food served at Café Yumm is very satisfying because it is prepared using fresh, quality ingredients and consistently tastes great. Food from Café Yumm is conveniently served in their restaurant or to go. Eating individual meals from large Yumm Bowls is very convenient. I enjoy them either as a whole meal or in smaller portions as a side dish with other foods that are part of my healthy eating program. I regularly add their sauces and salsas to various protein and vegetable dishes from my Healthy and Convenient Food List.

Restaurant: Chipotle Mexican Grill
Restaurant Type: Fast Service Healthy Mexican Grill
Prepared Foods I Eat or Take Home: Grilled marinated chicken, fajita vegetables
Health and Convenience: Chicken prepared and served at Chipotle Mexican Grill comes from chickens that were raised without antibiotics and fed a diet free of animal by-products. Grilled vegetables from Chipotle Mexican Grill are fresh sliced green peppers and red onions. I eat a single 4-oz. serving of grilled fajita chicken with a single 4-oz. serving of grilled vegetables as a part or all of one meal. I usually purchase a few servings of chicken and a few servings of vegetables at the same time and keep individual servings in my refrigerator. I enjoy Chipotle fajita chicken and grilled vegetables at home with an organic Haas avocado and organic blue corn chips on the side (avocado and chips are always available in my kitchen). This is another aspect of how I incorporate flexibility and convenience into my healthy eating program.

The Cost of Choosing to Eat Healthy

Many individual meals I consume are purchased from a restaurant or from a grocery store and usually cost $5.00 or less. There are exceptions. I occasionally eat leftovers from expensive restaurants, where the individual meal cost is higher. I also eat yogurt with trail mix and organic maple syrup where the individual meal cost is lower. Most of my meals are low cost because of portion control. Portion control is never forced because my body receives plenty of nutrients from the food I eat. Unless I am about to engage in vigorous exercise, my individual meal portion sizes are usually no larger than 7-8 ounces of food.

I vary my meal portions based on the level of exercise I have planned for the day and you should also!

Desserts and Sweets—Enjoy!

You will not stop eating sweet foods as part of your permanent healthy-eating program—don't even try; you will only set yourself up for failure! Remember, your "new" healthy-eating program is the healthy eating program you are going to be using for the rest of your life. Do not stop eating dessert! Apply the same principles that you are using with other foods and refrain from eating desserts that are loaded with highly processed ingredients. Instead, eat dessert treats made with minimally-processed and unprocessed ingredients and enjoy them without feeling guilty.

Throughout my 102-pound weight loss, I ate dessert treats every week. After two weeks on the Master Cleanse, I lost the desire to consume garbage foods, including sweets that contain substantial amounts of highly processed ingredients. The desserts I enjoyed during my weight loss and continue to eat today contain high-quality ingredients and are much more healthfully prepared than the desserts I used to eat (in much larger quantities). I usually try to only eat sweet foods if I know I will be engaging in intense exercise shortly afterward. If I eat dessert after dinner in the evening, I will typically have a strenuous work out planned the following morning.

My favorite desserts
- Cinnamon Red Maca Almond Butter from JEM Raw Chocolate
- Three Twins Organic Mint Confetti Ice Cream
- Organic Vegan Cupcakes from The Divine Cupcake

You might be very surprised by what you have just read. There is a very important concept to remember here. You are changing your life in order to lose weight and keep it off permanently! The healthy-eating program you will be on for the rest of your life MUST include indulgences or it won't work. You should not be surprised that after you successfully complete the Master Cleanse, you will be inclined to avoid highly processed foods and you WILL NOT have an issue with overeating—even sweets and desserts! I love Cinnamon Red Maca Almond Butter from JEM Raw Chocolate. I spread it on whole grain bread and also eat it with organic apples. You can find a variety of healthy indulgences from JEM Raw Chocolate in various grocery stores or order their products online at www.jemrawchocolate.com.

I also enjoy organic ice cream made by Three Twins. My favorite is Three Twins Mint Confetti Ice Cream that I purchase in one-pint sizes. I eat no more than one medium-size scoop and I still feel like I have enjoyed the complete experience of a sweet dessert. You can find Three Twins Ice Cream in various grocery stores or order it online at threetwinsicecream.com.

Locally in Eugene, I eat cupcakes from The Divine Cupcake. I usually only eat a small cupcake, particularly if I am enjoying it as dessert after a meal. I will indulge in a regular-size cupcake if I am headed out for a long run later in the day or evening.

The Takeaway
If your diet consists of nutrient-dense, minimally processed or unprocessed foods, you will not feel as though you are depriving yourself when you consume small portions of any type of food, including dessert.

Nutrition Bars: *A nutrition bar must be nutritious!*
There are many widely marketed, well-advertised "nutrition bars" that make the average consumer believe that they are eating a "much healthier version" of a candy bar. The most commonly used terms for these products are energy bars, protein bars, meal replacement bars, and nutrition bars. These products are a type of convenience food consumed primarily by people who are trying to lose weight.

The problem with many of these "healthier versions of candy bars" is they are completely detrimental to weight loss because they are highly processed, loaded with artificial ingredients, and contain substantial amounts of simple sugars and refined carbohydrates—making them as unhealthy as a commercially sold candy bar. There were many times during my overweight life that I ate these well-marketed products in futile attempts to lose weight.

Understanding food labels and avoiding highly processed foods whenever possible helped me choose a brand of nutrition bars that are actually nutritious. The nutrition bars I recommend are Picky Bars. I eat Picky Bars in conjunction with my exercise sessions or as snacks during the day. Picky Bars are made using wholesome, real ingredients and contain no artificial sweeteners. You can find Picky Bars online at www.pickybars.com.

Making the Healthier Choice

The concept that you can always make the healthiest food choice at any given time no matter where you are or what circumstance you find yourself in is completely un-realistic. There will be many occasions when you will need to make the healthier food choice. Opting for a healthier food choice when the healthiest food choice is not available will not mentally or emotionally derail your healthy lifestyle weight-loss program. The healthier choice should ALWAYS be analyzed from the perspective of nutrient content first—primarily focusing on avoiding highly processed food. Once you have analyzed the nutrient content, focus on the macronutrients that the product contains (grams of protein, carbs, and fats).

Healthier Choice Example

Let's assume you are traveling and are in an unfamiliar town. The probability that you will always be able to locate the healthiest restaurant (assuming there is one) serving only organic wholesome food is next to zero. If you are able to find such a restaurant, the probability that you will be able to eat every meal there is also next to zero. Based on your circumstances, you should always default to the healthier choice.

Eat *Two Moms in the Raw Granola*, Simply Nuts and Fruit Snacks, Peeled Snacks, or a Protein Bistro Box if it is available at a Starbucks. Don't eat pre-packaged, highly processed burritos, cheeseburgers, or deli packs purchased from a gas station. When I purchase a healthy food box, I don't feel like I have to eat everything in the box so that I can "get my money's worth." I eat the best items from the box and discard the rest.

A Healthier Way to Enjoy an Unhealthy Indulgence

There is always a healthier way to enjoy what is otherwise considered to be an unhealthy meal. To illustrate this I offer the cheeseburger and fries example.

Healthier Example of a Cheeseburger and Fries

The healthier version of a cheeseburger can either be eaten without a bun or on a whole grain bun. A cheeseburger prepared using an organic beef burger (beef from cows raised on grass never having been given antibiotics, added hormones, or animal by-products) topped with a slice of organic or natural cheese (rBGH-free), organic vegetables (vegetables not sprayed with chemicals and pesticides), and organic condiments (condiments not containing highly processed ingredients) accompanied by a side of baked sweet potato fries is the healthier example of a cheeseburger and fries. The healthy ingredients in this example are as easy to acquire and the meal is as easy to prepare as the unhealthy version you have probably been eating for years.

Important Guidelines for Weight Loss Related to a Permanent Healthy-Eating Program

- Consume a diet of nutrient-rich, unprocessed or minimally processed foods.
- Consume substantial amounts of protein throughout the day relative to carbohydrates and fats.
- Consume healthy complex carbohydrates sourced primarily from organic fruits and vegetables.
- Consume a minimal amount of sugar—always all natural or organic and never refined.
- Consume a minimum of five small meals each day.
- Drink a minimum amount of water each day that equals in ounces your current body weight in pounds divided in half.

**Important Guidelines for Conveniently
Incorporating Healthy Eating into Your Life**

- Healthy food must be accessible to you at all times.
- Always have food available that can be conveniently prepared and assembled into a meal in seven minutes or less.
- Do not feel obligated to eat the same meal as other members of your family even if you are eating with them.
- Don't limit your individual choices by eating only breakfast foods for breakfast, lunch foods for lunch, or dinner foods for dinner. Be amenable to eating any foods that are part of your healthy eating program at any time during the day to accommodate your circumstance (feel free to enjoy a quinoa salad early in the morning and high-protein Greek yogurt with trail mix and organic maple syrup in the evening). Eating for convenience works so long as your body receives the nutrients it needs!

Chapter SEVEN

A CONVENIENT EXERCISE PROGRAM FOR EXTREME WEIGHT LOSS

The Importance of Exercise

One of the lifestyle changes that my weight-loss program requires is a commitment to weekly exercise. Exercise will play an essential role in your immediate weight loss and future weight maintenance and should not be discontinued once you lose your desired amount of weight. When we get older, we lose muscle mass. When muscle mass is lost, our metabolism slows down. When our metabolism slows down, we burn fewer calories. The fewer calories we burn, the more weight we are likely to gain. Exercising on a regular basis enables the metabolism to be consistently stimulated, which burns calories. Eating nutrient-rich food and performing strength-training and cardiovascular exercises (cardio) will ensure the success of immediate weight loss and future weight maintenance.

A Fundamental Knowledge of Exercise

Weight and Strength Training

Weight training is a form of strength training and is absolutely critical to the success of any weight-loss and weight-maintenance program. Primarily, weight training raises the metabolism—muscle burns more calories than fat. Most people who visit a health club for the first time find the weight room to be very intimidating.

You should never feel like you want to throw your hands up and quit your workout program because you are confused or unmotivated. The more difficult your exercise program is to understand, the more likely you are to quit. You need to walk confidently into your health club and know that you are using a strength-training program that you will be able to follow consistently! In this chapter you will find the strength-training program that I created for myself. I utilized a circuit-training workout program to lose my excess weight and continue to use the same program to maintain my healthy weight.

There are many people that show up at my gym each year on January 1, committed to the idea of losing weight as part of their annual New Year's resolution. Unfortunately but not surprisingly, many stop showing up after a couple of weeks. The reason for this is they become uncomfortable in their surroundings, unmotivated by their program, and unsure of the benefits that they are receiving as a result of their hard work. Numerous individuals attempt to engage in exercise that is far beyond their physical capabilities.

My strength-training program will never put you in an "extreme boot camp" situation where you are miserable and physically sick after your workouts.

A solid strength-training program will allow you to step off of the high-speed-weight-gain locomotive with confidence and leap on to the healthy-weight-loss-and-future-weight-maintenance locomotive headed in the opposite direction on an endless track. Put another way, the exercise portion of my weight-loss program is designed to be realistic and sustainable for people who want to lose weight quickly and keep it off permanently.

Understanding Strength Training
In order to have a successful strength-training session, your muscles must be engaged. There must be resistance for muscles to be engaged. If there is no resistance, there is no benefit. In order to achieve the maximum benefit from strength training, we must use correct form. Never walk into the gym and mindlessly use equipment as if you are going through the motions. Decide how you are going to move before engaging in each exercise. Performing strength-training exercises

using correct form is very important. If correct form is not used, most of the effectiveness of a strength-training workout is lost.

Strength training using correct form includes the following:
- Use the full range of motion intended for each specific exercise.
- Use resistance and not momentum during each exercise. Pushing, pulling, lifting, and lowering movements should be performed in a controlled fashion without using a swinging or jerking motion during the exercise.
- Breathe consistently during each exercise.

Use Circuit-Training to Complete Strength-Training Workouts
Circuit training is the most convenient, efficient, and effective way to complete strength-training workouts. I used circuit training throughout my 102-pound weight loss to complete my strength-training workouts and I continue to use circuit-training workouts to maintain my healhty weight to this day!

In order to circuit train properly, each exercise in the circuit is completed one right after the other during a rotation with little or no break in-between. No less than four and no more than five exercises are completed during each circuit-training rotation. Do not rest more than two to three minutes between each completed circuit-training rotation. When you complete a total of four circuit-training rotations, you have completed a full strength-training workout.

A Complete Strength-Training Workout
- 4-5 exercises = 1 rotation
- Little or no break between each exercise
- 2-3 minute break between each rotation
- 4 total rotations = 1 complete strength-training workout session

Cardiovascular Exercise (Cardio)

In addition to strength training, cardio is another key component to successful weight loss and future weight maintenance. Cardio exercise will increase your metabolism, which is essential for weight loss and weight maintenance. The heart is a muscle; it needs to be exercised in order to be healthy and strong.

People usually fall into two different groups when it comes to cardiovascular exercise. One group includes people who find cardio exercises boring, repetitive, and a waste of time. The other group includes people who love cardio exercise. Many formerly overweight people become passionate about a particular type of cardio that helped facilitate their weight loss.

One of the biggest challenges related to weight loss and weight maintenance is helping people move from the bored group to the motivated group. You will find that your continued weight loss is a powerful motivator to sustain your exercise program. When I decided to lose my excess weight and keep it off permanently, I knew that it would be imperative for me to view cardiovascular exercise differently than I had before (I used to be in the first group). The mental aspect of weight loss will always facilitate the physical aspect of weight loss.

Viewing Cardio Differently

Cardio typically consists of walking, running, biking, swimming, elliptical machine, and rowing machine exercises. Cardio exercises may also be accomplished in specialized classes such as spinning and kickboxing at fitness facilities that offer them. You must choose at least two or more types of cardio exercises that you are prepared to use in your program to help facilitate your weight loss—it is important to vary your workouts. I initially chose the elliptical machine, seated stationary bike, and treadmill (walking on the treadmill—I walked because I was not able to run on the treadmill when I began my final weight loss at 271 pounds).

Beginning a cardio program is initially depressing when you are significantly overweight like I was because you cannot believe how out of shape you are, especially if you are comparing your current fitness level to a different time in your life when you used to be fit. Do not get discouraged! You will discover that when you stick with your cardio workouts, you will quickly become more physically fit. Within a few weeks of exercise, you will not believe how quickly you have advanced relative to where you began. This is very empowering and will give you the constant mental push to proceed with your weight loss.

Once you are consistently engaged in cardiovascular exercise, you will discover that it is a great time for you to tune the rest of the world out and focus on your own thoughts. I love the time I spend doing my cardio and find it to be mentally and physically uplifting.

I listen to music on my iPod and tune out the rest of the world during my cardio exercise. I have found that cardio gives me a lot of serenity and I never dread it or view it as a chore. You might discover that you enjoy your cardio workouts if you approach it this same way.

Alternatively, you might find that joining an aerobics class and working out with a group of people in the same challenging setting is appealing to you. Find cardio exercises that you enjoy doing so that you are able to sustain your weight loss.

Focusing on the Goal
The primary goal for any overweight person starting an exercise program should be to lose weight.

- In order to incorporate a successful exercise program into your weight-loss regimen, it must be convenient. You must be able to achieve maximum benefit in a convenient amount of time. When an exercise program becomes inconvenient, it ceases to exist and weight-loss failure is initiated.
- Your exercise program must be easy to understand. By design, my exercise program is very easy to understand and follow on a continual basis.

- Most importantly, your exercise program must be effective. An exercise program that is not effective is completely worthless.

People stick with exercise programs because they are seeing results. I saw extraordinary results while I was on my weight-loss program because I successfully implemented my exercise program with my healthy eating program.

Creating an effective workout program that everyone can use to lose weight

My program is designed for anyone and everyone who has a desire to lose weight—the everyman and everywoman. Put another way, everyone should be able to lose weight by consistently sticking with an exercise program that is convenient, effective, and easy to understand. My exercise program is not designed to turn you into a professional body builder or an Olympic athlete. My exercise program is designed to enable you to significantly improve your health, increase your fitness level at a consistent pace, lose weight quickly, and live the rest of your life as someone who has taken off their excess weight permanently.

The 5-95 Weight-Loss Exercise Program

My strength-training/cardio weight-loss and weight-maintenance program is called the 5-95 Weight-Loss Exercise Program. It is sometimes referred to in this chapter and on my website as 5-95. The 5 in 5-95 relates to committing approximately 5% of the total hours each week to exercise. The 95 in 5-95 relates to the fact that if you spend 5% of your week exercising, you will spend the other 95% of your week looking and feeling great (coincidentally I lost 95 pounds in one year on my program).

What happens when you commit 5% of the hours in your week to exercise?

- You will lose all of the weight and body fat you need to lose.
- You will improve your overall health immeasurably and reduce your risk of cardiovascular and other deadly diseases.
- You will set yourself up for being able to maintain a healthy weight for the rest of your life.

Weekly Exercise Goals

Weekly exercise goals work. Daily and monthly exercise goals don't work and are a set-up for failure. The reasons are simple. Daily exercise goals don't work because life gets in the way (your child has to go to the doctor, you get called out of town on work, your car breaks down). Should one of life's inconveniences present itself, your daily workout program is derailed. Monthly exercise goals are too hard to keep track of and encourage procrastination. Weekly workout goals are easily tracked and much easier to adhere to than daily or monthly workout goals!

> **IMPORTANT:** I used the Master Cleanse for two weeks and spent three days coming off of it. I exercised during the first 13 days I was on the cleanse. I did not adhere to the time requirements in the 5-95 Weight-Loss Exercise Program until my fourth week of weight loss. I familiarized myself with circuit-training exercises as part of my strength-training program and completed as much cardio exercise as possible while I was committed to the Master Cleanse. I was able to complete my weekly exercise requirements on my fourth week of weight loss once I emerged from the Master Cleanse. Ideally, you should be able to complete the weekly requirements included in 5-95 no later than the beginning of your fifth week of weight loss.

Do not get discouraged if you need more time to build up to the exercise requirements of 5-95, everyone starts at a different place. Where you start is not important—where you finish is everything!

Beginning Your Weight-Loss Program with an Existing Injury

If you have an existing injury when you start my final weight-loss program, you must choose exercises that do not make your injury worse. For example, if you begin your weight loss with an existing knee injury, you will probably not want to choose running on the treadmill as one of your cardio options. You might choose swimming instead—perhaps only moving your upper body while keeping your injured knee stationary. My exercise program is flexible—there are many different types of cardio exercise that will facilitate your weight loss. Always be focused on your goal, which is staying on the weight-loss program.

Completing the 5-95 Cardio Weekly Requirement

In order to fulfill the 5-95 weekly cardio requirements, you must complete a minimum of five hours of moderately intense gym or gym-equivalent cardio each week using a minimum of two different types of cardiovascular exercises. Feel free to choose different cardio machines and exercises as part of your own program (running, elliptical, biking, swimming, aerobics class, etc.). You must feel a challenge from your cardio workout and it must raise your heart rate.

You will discover that as your cardio fitness improves, your level of moderate intensity will increase. The distance you choose to travel down the path of cardio fitness will be up to you and what your desired goals become once you have lost your weight. Ultimately you might engage in interval training cardio workouts because you are at an advanced level of exercising. You should not try to engage in difficult, complicated, and confusing workout programs when you begin your final weight loss because you won't be able to maintain it. Remember, your goal is to stick with your program and your immediate focus is weight loss. Do not engage in high-intensity exercise on a consistent basis when you first start your weight-loss program. You must build up your endurance and not put yourself at risk of getting an injury.

Consistency is the most important aspect of exercise and weight loss!

The 5-95 Strength-Training Weekly Requirements

In order to fulfill the 5-95 weekly strength-training requirements, you must complete a minimum of three strength-training sessions per week. Each strength-training session can be completed in approximately 35 minutes.

Weight-training exercises are part of your strength-training program. During your weight-training exercises, you should lift approximately 65-70% of the maximum weight you are capable of lifting one time (referred to here as your max).

Strength-Training Weight-Loss Exercises

A complete circuit-training rotation is composed of four or five exercises that include pushing exercises, pulling exercises, lower body dominant exercises, and core exercises. **Fifteen repetitions** should be completed during each exercise. To reiterate, no less than four and no more than five exercises should be completed in one rotation. Four completed circuit-training rotations equals one strength-training session.

Example of One Complete Circuit-Training Rotation Using 5-95 Exercises

Pushing Exercise:	Incline Bench Press	15 Repetitions
Pulling Exercise:	Narrow Grip Lat Pull-Down	15 Repetitions
Lower Body Dominant Exercise:	Combined Exercise Including Leg Press and Leg Curl	15 Repetitions Each
Core Exercise:	Plank	Hold 15 Seconds

Completing 15 repetitions of each exercise = 1 rotation
Completing 4 total rotations = 1 completed strength-training workout

Important Information Before You Get Started

- Beginners should use machines instead of free weights whenever possible. Machines are easier to use and highly effective. When you become more comfortable with lifting weights, you can incorporate free weights into your workouts if you choose.
- I highly recommend purchasing a minimum of three personal training sessions at your health club when you first get started. A qualified trainer will guide you through the circuit exercises I recommend in this chapter to ensure that you are using correct form. Tell your trainer that you are using circuit-training exercise rotations that include pushing exercises, pulling exercises, lower body dominant exercises, and core exercises in each rotation. The specific exercises listed in this chapter should be given to your trainer so he or she can show you the correct way to perform each exercise. You should not need more than three personal training sessions to understand how to correctly perform all of the exercises.
- Remember to use controlled movements during your strength-training workouts. Never lift weights using a jerking motion.
- Remember to breathe during your strength-training exercises. Do not hold your breath. Be in control!

I have included some instruction with the recommended exercises in the 5-95 Weight-Loss Exercise Program. There is an abundance of valuable free information (including pictures and instructional videos) about the exercises I recommend that can be easily found on the internet by entering the name of the exercise into a search engine. I do not want to inundate you with pages of written instruction here because it is not realistic to assume that you will carry this book around with you in your health club. The easiest and most efficient way to get started is to know what the exercises are, grasp a general understanding of how each exercise is used in circuit-training format, and use the services of a knowledgeable personal trainer so that you can learn how to perform the exercises correctly.

The following exercise recommendations for each individual circuit category (including pushing, pulling, lower body dominant, and core exercises) are designed for you to achieve maximum benefit from your strength training and ensure that you are able to consistently perform the exercises in the 5-95 Weight-Loss Exercise Program each week. You are not expected to limit yourself to these specific exercises forever. There are many pushing, pulling, lower-body dominant, and core exercises for you incorporate into your strength-training workouts in the future. The exercises I have listed here are highly effective exercises to get you started down the path of weight loss. You can choose from any of the exercises options that I list in each category so long as you vary your choices (don't use the same strength-training routine back to back during the week).

I designed my circuit-training workouts so that each strength-training session will always be efficient. Consistent exercise must be convenient in your life—just like eating healthy must be convenient in your life! Let's assume you happen to go to the gym during a busy time; your 35-minute workout should not take you an hour and a half to complete because the gym is crowded! You can choose from multiple exercises within each individual circuit category on the list—some exercises involve using your own body weight as resistance instead of a machine. This will make your circuit training much more efficient because you will not be waiting around for machines to become available.

PUSHING EXERCISES

A pushing exercise is defined as pushing weight away from the body.

Best Exercise Choices for the 5-95 Weight-Loss Exercise Program:
- Incline Chest Press (15 repetitions each circuit rotation)
- Push Up (15 repetitions each circuit rotation)

The incline chest press and push-up exercises are the pushing exercise choices in the 5-95 Weight-Loss Exercise Program. Each exercise is highly effective and can be conveniently performed in most fitness facilities.

Incline Chest Press:

Primary muscles engaged: chest (upper), deltoids (anterior), triceps

Benefit:

The incline chest press is highly effective because you are heavily engaging three different muscle groups with one exercise.

Convenience:

The incline chest press can be performed by using dumbbells or an incline chest press machine, which makes it very convenient as part of a circuit-training workout, particularly if the gym is crowded and you are moving from exercise to exercise.

IMPORTANT: Beginners should use a machine instead of dumbbells whenever possible.

Push Up

Primary muscles engaged: chest (upper), deltoids, serratus, cora-cobrachialis, triceps

Benefit:

Push-up exercises are highly effective because you are heavily engaging five different muscle groups with one exercise.

Convenience:

Push-up exercises are very convenient. You can tailor the push-up to meet your fitness and strength levels because you are using your own body weight as resistance. Push-ups can be performed from many different starting positions. You can change angular positions to make the exercise more or less challenging. If you are extremely overweight or physically compromised like I was, you can start your push-up motion with your knees on the ground—a much easier position than starting with your feet on the ground. The push-up exercise can also be completed by using a pushing motion against a firm elevated surface such as a wall or high ledge.

PULLING EXERCISES
A pulling exercise is defined as pulling weight toward the body.

Best Exercise Choices for 5-95 Weight-Loss Exercise Program
- Seated cable row (15 repetitions each circuit rotation)
- Narrow grip lat pull-down (15 repetitions each circuit rotation)
- Assisted pull-up (15 repetitions each circuit rotation)

The seated cable row, narrow grip lat pull-down, and assisted pull-up exercises are the chosen pulling exercise choices in the 5-95 Weight-Loss Exercise Workout Program. Each exercise is highly effective and can be conveniently accomplished in most fitness facilities.

Seated Cable Row
Primary muscles engaged: back (mainly latissimus dorsi [lats]), deltoids (posterior), biceps

Benefit:
You are heavily engaging three different muscle groups with one exercise.

Convenience:
The Seated Cable Row exercise is always performed using a machine. Every health club that has a weight room should have a seated cable row machine. Many hotels and motels that offer an exercise facility with weights have a seated cable row machine.

Narrow Grip Lat Pull-Down
Primary muscles engaged: back (lats), biceps, shoulders

Benefit:
Although the narrow grip lat pull-down exercise primarily engages the lat muscles located on either side of the middle of the back, the biceps and shoulders also receive a great workout from this exercise.

Convenience:
The narrow grip lat pull-down exercise is always performed using a machine. Every health club that has a weight room should have a lat pull-down machine. Many hotels and motels that offer an exercise facility with weights will also have a lat pull-down machine.

Assisted Pull-Up
Primary muscles engaged: back (mainly lats, trapezius [traps], and rhomboid muscles)

Benefit:
You are heavily engaging your middle and upper back muscles with one exercise.

Convenience:
The assisted pull-up exercise can be specifically tailored to meet your strength levels. The assisted pull-up machine allows you to either kneel on a pad or stand on a platform and use a weight machine stack to assist you during your movement.

> **IMPORTANT:** Beginners should start with a weight stack using approximately 15 pounds less than their body weight. Use less weight on the assisted stack to lift more body weight as fitness levels improve. Additionally, the more weight you continue to lose, the less weight you will need on the assisted stack!

LOWER BODY DOMINANT EXERCISES

Lower body dominant exercises work the muscles in the lower body. Most people who go to a gym focus primarily on upper body muscles during their strength-training sessions. The leg muscles should not be ignored in your workout routine as they are an integral part of strength-training workouts. The muscles in your legs represent some of the largest muscles in your body (remember, the more muscle mass you have, the more calories you burn—exercising your largest muscles will help you lose weight).

Best Exercise Choices for 5-95 Weight-Loss Exercise Program:

- Sit to stand (also known as sit and stand—15 repetitions each circuit rotation)
- Leg press/leg curl combination as one exercise (15 repetitions each during the same circuit rotation)

The sit to stand and leg press/leg curl exercises are the lower body dominant exercise choices in the 5-95 Weight-Loss Exercise Program. Each exercise is highly effective and can be conveniently accomplished in most fitness facilities. When you are using the leg press/leg curl combination in your circuit rotation, you should always perform the leg press first. You will complete a total of five exercises during your circuit-training rotation when you use the leg press and leg curl machines as your lower body dominant exercise. When you perform the sit-to-stand exercise, you will complete a total of four exercises during your circuit-training rotation.

Sit to Stand

Primary muscles engaged: quadriceps (quads), hamstrings, gluteus maximus and gluteus minimus (glutes), calves, tibialis

Benefit:

You are heavily engaging five different lower body muscle groups with one exercise. Sit to stand is mostly thought of as a functional movement to get up and down. Performed in repetition, it is an exercise that is essentially a form of a squat.

Convenience:
Sit to stand exercises can be performed most places in your health club where a flat seated bench surface is available. You can tailor the sit to stand exercise to meet your fitness and strength levels because you can use your hands to assist with the movement.

IMPORTANT: Do not mindlessly sit down and stand up 15 times to perform this exercise. Use a slow, controlled specific motion starting with your heels a few inches in front of the bench you are sitting on. Your feet should be lined up a little wider than shoulder width apart and your toes should be slightly turned out. You can lightly assist with your hands on top of each thigh to help with balance and lifting your body weight off of the bench if needed. Keep your eyes forward, chin slightly up, and shoulders slightly back. Ease back on the bench and stand using another slow controlled movement. When you sit back down, you should immediately stand up when you feel contact with the flat surface. Repeat 15 times as one exercise during your circuit.

Leg Press/Leg Curl Combination
Primary muscles engaged:
Leg press: quads, glutes, hamstrings
Leg curl: hamstrings

Specific Instructions:
The leg press exercise should be performed first during the lower body dominant portion of your circuit training rotation, then the leg curl exercise (each exercise uses a different machine).

Benefit:
You are heavily engaging different lower body dominant muscle groups during each individual circuit-training rotation.

Convenience:

Leg press and leg curl exercises are performed using machines. Using different machines during the same circuit-training workout will allow you to work more muscle groups during one strength-training session.

CORE EXERCISES

Core exercises are essential for improving balance and stability, strengthening abdominal and back muscles, and minimizing overall risk of injury. Core exercises are some of the more important exercises for continued health and well-being.

Best Exercise Choices for 5-95 Weight-Loss Exercise Program

- Plank (hold for 15 seconds each circuit rotation)
- Bird dog (extend both sets of opposite limbs 15 times each circuit rotation)
- Reverse crunch (15 repetitions each circuit rotation)

Plank, bird-dog, and reverse crunch exercises are the chosen exercises in the 5-95 Weight-Loss Exercise Program. Each exercise is highly effective and can be conveniently accomplished in most fitness facilities.

Plank

Primary muscles engaged: abdominal, lower back

Benefit:

Plank is a great exercise that enables you to strengthen two major muscle groups in your core region.

Convenience:

No equipment is required to engage in the plank exercise. You are only using your body weight and gravity as resistance.

Specific Instructions:

Your upper body should be supported by your forearms on an elevated cushioned bench. Your legs will be on an even plane with your upper body with your feet on the floor balancing on your toes, which are shoulder width apart. Your body should be in alignment from your shoulders to your ankles. Tighten your abdominal muscles and lower back while still continuing to breathe. Hold the tightened position while the body remains motionless throughout the plank exercise. Instead of 15 repetitions, hold for a minimum of fifteen seconds without breaking form. One way to advance in the plank exercise is to hold your position for a longer period of time without breaking form. Another method you can use to achieve a more challenging plank exercise is to perform the exercise with your feet closer together. You can always make your plank exercise more difficult as you become more advanced in your strength training.

Bird Dog
Primary muscles engaged: lower back, abdominal, glutes

Benefit:
The benefit of the bird-dog exercise is to strengthen the lower back muscles in order to prevent injury. You are strengthening three different muscle groups with one exercise.

Convenience:
No equipment is required to engage in the bird-dog exercise.

> **Specific Instructions:**
> Make sure there is plenty of cushion supporting your knees while performing this exercise (foam exercise pads work great and can be found in most fitness facilities). The more overweight you are, the more your knees will need to be supported.

Kneel on all fours and start with your arms and thighs perpendicular to the floor. Your hands and knees should be shoulder width apart. Your back should be flat and your spine should be straight. While keeping your spine straight, extend opposite limbs at the same time (the left leg extends straight out from the hip and the right arm extends straight out from the shoulder—hold for two seconds and return to start position— then the right leg extends straight out from the hip and left arm extends straight out from the shoulder—hold for two seconds and return to start position). Make sure your hips and back remain parallel to the floor (without any rotation of the hip) the entire time while performing the exercise (if a ball was placed in the small of your back it wouldn't fall off during the exercise movement). You must remember to breathe while performing the bird-dog exercise. Your core should be engaged throughout the entire movement. One repetition has been completed when both sets of opposite limbs have been extended. Complete a total of 15 repetitions in each circuit-training rotation.

Reverse Crunch
Primary muscles engaged: rectus abdominis, transversus abdominis

Benefit:
In addition to engaging two major abdominal muscle groups, reverse crunch exercises will also engage your oblique muscles.

Convenience:
Other than a mat or comfortable floor surface, no equipment is required to engage in a reverse crunch exercise.

Specific Instructions:
Lie on your back on a comfortable floor surface or exercise mat. Place your hands and arms flat on the floor alongside your body. Keep your eyes on the ceiling without bending your neck while performing this exercise. While making sure your abs are tightened and pulled toward your spine, lift your legs and bend your knees to 90 degrees. Using a controlled, deliberate motion, pull your knees toward your chest and hold the position for two seconds. Lower your legs back to the starting position using a controlled, deliberate motion to complete one repetition.

IMPORTANT: You may place your hands on your posterior thigh muscles and gently pull to assist with the reverse crunch exercise.

Important Guidelines for a Consistent Exercise Program

- The most important aspect of my 5-95 Weight-Loss Exercise Program is to be consistent and complete your weekly workout requirements.

- Do not get discouraged, particularly when you begin your final weight-loss program. Your starting fitness level is what it is; you cannot change the past. You must look forward to what will be your incredible life transformation in the future.

- There will be occasions when your cardio session is easy and you struggle during your strength-training session. There will be other occasions when your strength-training session is easy and you struggle during your cardio session. There will be days when both are more difficult than usual. Do not get discouraged—being committed to your weekly exercise program on a consistent basis is what will enable you to lose weight!

- Do not be overzealous and risk injury when you start your workout program. Being sore after a workout is acceptable and expected. Sustaining an injury could hinder the progression of your weight loss.

- Always drink plenty of water before, during, and after your workouts.

Summary

The 5-95 Weight Loss Exercise Program is designed to be convenient, easy to implement, and very effective.

The strength-training exercises in the 5-95 Weight-Loss Exercise Program can be used in any respectable health club. I traveled extensively for work while I was losing weight and stayed in different hotels and motels that had extremely limited fitness facilities and was still able to complete my weekly exercise requirements. My confidence levels soared each week as I got in better shape and continued to lose weight. Your confidence levels will soar also!

Chapter EIGHT

THE FIRST 21 DAYS

This chapter will provide you with a general guide to help you get started down the path of weight loss. You are not expected to replicate the exact events of my first three weeks of weight loss. Use the suggestions and information as a helpful guide and incorporate your own routine that best fits your lifestyle. I completed all of my preliminary weight-loss preparations on a Sunday and began my weight loss on a Monday. I highly recommend that you do the same.

Do not expect to accomplish all aspects of my 5-95 Weight-Loss Exercise Program while you are using the Master Cleanse. Use your time on the Master Cleanse the way I used mine. Join a health club if you are not already a member of one and complete a minimum of three strength trainings sessions (low-intensity) with a qualified personal trainer. Your personal training sessions will enable you to familiarize yourself with the strength-training exercises in my 5-95 Weight-Loss Exercise Program. Begin low-intensity cardiovascular exercise (e.g., low to moderate speed on a treadmill, low to moderate intensity using an elliptical machine). You will lose a significant amount of weight while you are on the Master Cleanse. Do not burden yourself with intense workouts to enhance your weight loss while on the cleanse.

If you start to cramp or feel light-headed during your workout session while you are on the Master Cleanse, discontinue exercise for the day and drink more Master Cleanse Mixture immediately! If you decide to use a different cleanse, apply the same general principles.

The Day Before You Officially Start Your Final Weight Loss
Purchase all items you will need to begin the Master Cleanse including a gallon jug for your mixture and a large container for your water. Buy enough ingredients to last most of the first week on the cleanse (enjoy the scent of lemon in your kitchen).

Make sure that you are all set to conveniently walk in and use your chosen health club (membership paperwork completed and current, appointments established with a personal trainer). You should be able to arrive on your first day of your weight-loss program and get started immediately.

GO TIME!

DAY 1

- Wake up, use the bathroom, and weigh yourself.
- Document your starting weight.
- Prepare an 80-ounce or larger mixture of the Master Cleanse Recipe in a one-gallon jug—remember not to include the cayenne tincture (add separately to each 10-oz. serving—two individual drops per serving). Drink your first serving and continue to drink the mixture throughout the day.
- Drink 8 ounces of water and continue to drink water throughout the day.
- Go to your health club when it is convenient. Walk on the treadmill for a maximum of 15 minutes. Complete a light elliptical workout for a maximum of 15 minutes.
- Drink a serving of Traditional Medicinals Smooth Move Tea before bed.

Highlights from My Day 1:

Only my wife and one of our friends knew I was starting the Master Cleanse. I woke up, used the bathroom, and weighed myself—271 pounds. I prepared the Master Cleanse Mixture and drank three cups during the morning before arriving at the gym at noon. I walked into Gold's Gym in Eugene, Oregon, flashed my membership card, and immediately went upstairs to the cardio machines.

I was clearly the heaviest and most out-of-shape person in the gym. This did not matter to me because I had already mentally prepared myself not to get discouraged. Being the heaviest person at the gym meant I would have the greatest story to tell once I lost all of my weight! I completed 15 minutes on the elliptical machine, 15 minutes on the treadmill, and made a mental note to apply Vaseline to the insides of my legs before future cardio exercises. My thighs were so large, they rubbed together and chaffed during my cardio session. Everyone has to start someplace.

DAY 2

- Wake up, use the bathroom, and weigh yourself.
- Prepare your Master Cleanse Mixture. Drink your first serving and continue to drink the mixture throughout the day.
- Drink 8 ounces of water and continue to drink water throughout the day.
- Go to your health club when it is convenient. Exercise on a stationary bicycle machine for a maximum of 15 minutes. Complete your first circuit strength-training workout using a personal trainer.

Highlights from My Day 2:

I woke up and weighed myself—269 pounds. Under 270 pounds—a small accomplishment noted! I drank two cups of the Master Cleanse Mixture and accompanied Lisa to Creswell Coffee. This would be my first true test of will power. Why would I do this when I was only on my second day of the cleanse? I knew I would be constantly tested during the first two weeks—I might as well get the first big one out of the way.

Melissa (one of the owners of Creswell Coffee) looked at me with a curious stare when I told her that I was not ordering my usual, a 16-oz. latte with two Equal Sweeteners and a Raisin Danish. Melissa became the next person to learn that I was on the Master Cleanse. I drank two large cups of water and watched Lisa enjoy a danish and a 16-oz. mocha. I went to Gold's Gym in the afternoon and completed my first strength-training workout. Following my strength-training workout, I applied Vaseline to the insides of my thighs and completed a 15-minute cardio session on a seated stationary bike.

DAY 3

- Wake up, use the bathroom, and weigh yourself.
- Prepare your Master Cleanse Mixture. Drink your first serving and continue to drink the mixture throughout the day.
- Drink 8 ounces of water and continue to drink water throughout the day.
- Go to your health club when it is convenient. Complete one or two low-intensity 15-minute cardio sessions (exercise machines of your choice).
- Drink a serving of Traditional Medicinals Smooth Move Tea before bed.

Highlights from My Day 3:

I woke up and weighed myself—266 pounds. I drank two servings of the Master Cleanse Mixture and immediately went to the gym and completed a 15-minute walk on the treadmill and a 15-minute elliptical exercise. While on the treadmill, I remembered that I had forgotten to apply Vaseline to the inside of my thighs and chaffed my legs again. Apparently my short-term memory does not last 46 hours. Lesson finally learned! I took a nap late in the afternoon. Lisa walked in the bedroom while I was asleep and thought I had died because I was not snoring. When she leaned over to check on me, she heard me breathing peacefully—taking long, deep breaths. Unbeknownst to either of us at the time, I had permanently stopped snoring.

DAY 4

- Wake up, use the bathroom, and weigh yourself.
- Prepare your Master Cleanse Mixture. Drink your first serving and continue to drink the mixture throughout the day.
- Drink 8 ounces of water and continue to drink water throughout the day.
- Go to your health club when it is convenient and complete your second circuit-training workout using a personal training session.

NOTE: Some of my friends and family members used the Master Cleanse once they saw how well it worked for me. Most of them started having a very difficult time with it when they reached Day 4. Hang in there—your results will be fantastic if you stay on the program!

Highlights from My Day 4:

My water container had become my new best friend. Water was always immediately accessible to me while I was on the cleanse. I found myself constantly using the restroom. I did not view this as an imposition because I desperately needed to eliminate the toxins I had accumulated in my body as a result of eating a garbage diet for so many years. The Traditional Medicinals Smooth Move Tea was doing its job—no need to elaborate further on that topic!

DAY 5

- Wake up, use the bathroom, and weigh yourself.
- Prepare your Master Cleanse Mixture. Drink your first serving and continue to drink the mixture throughout the day.
- Drink 8 ounces of water and continue to drink water throughout the day.
- Go to your health club when it is convenient. Complete a light circuit-training workout on your own. Remember to make controlled movements during your strength-training session. Make mental notes of things you are unsure about so that you can address them in your next personal training session.
- Drink a serving of Traditional Medicinals Smooth Move Tea before bed.

Highlights from My Day 5:

I woke up and weighed myself—262.5 pounds. I could not believe that I was already within days of being in the 250s. I drank a few servings of the Master Cleanse Mixture throughout the morning and went to the gym around 2 PM. I completed a strength-training workout, drove home, felt a slight headache coming on, and took two Advil. Lisa mentioned to me that evening that my weight loss was starting to become noticeable. I knew she was being sincere—this was not the love talking! I was ecstatic given that I was only five days into my program.

DAY 6

- Wake up, use the bathroom, and weigh yourself.
- Prepare your Master Cleanse Mixture. Drink your first serving and continue to drink the mixture throughout the day.
- Drink 8 ounces of water and continue to drink water throughout the day.
- Take the day off from going to your health club.
- Go to the grocery store and replenished your supplies if you haven't already.

Highlights from My Day 6:

I woke up on Day 6 and immediately noticed how deeply I was breathing. My air passages were wide open. My muscles were sore from strength training and I remember being able to actually feel my own weight loss for the first time. I weighed 261 pounds—10 pounds lost, more to come! I drank a couple of servings of the Master Cleanse Mixture, grabbed my water container, and went to the grocery store to replenish lemons and Grade B dark amber maple syrup. I was starting to get used to drinking a gallon of water a day.

DAY 7

- Wake up, use the bathroom, and weigh yourself.
- Prepare your Master Cleanse Mixture. Drink your first serving and continue to drink the mixture throughout the day.
- Drink 8 ounces of water and continue to drink water throughout the day.
- Go to your health club when it is convenient. Complete a 30-minute low-intensity cardio exercise on the machine of your choice.
- Drink a serving of Traditional Medicinals Smooth Move Tea before bed.

Congratulations! One week down. You have made a commitment to health and weight loss! You will continue to be rewarded. There are much greater things that will come your way. Hang in there!

IMPORTANT: Remember to keep drinking substantial amounts of water.

Highlights from My Day 7:
I woke up, used the bathroom, and weighed myself—I was still 261 pounds, which I found hard to believe considering the fact that I was peeing like a broken fire hydrant. I was not discouraged because I did not expect to lose weight every day. The only expectation I had placed on myself was to stick with my program. I drank multiple servings of Master Cleanse Mixture in the morning and left for the gym at 1 PM.

Although I had only been exercising for a week, on Day 7 I realized that my cardio had improved dramatically. I easily completed a 30-minute medium-intensity cardio session on the elliptical machine. Day 7 was the day I started to view cardio differently. I discovered that I thoroughly enjoyed listening to music on my iPod and being in my own world during my cardio workouts. The muscle pain I experienced from my strength-training sessions felt rewarding, and I began to look forward to strength-training.

DAY 8

- Wake up, use the bathroom, and weigh yourself.
- Prepare your Master Cleanse Mixture. Drink your first serving and continue to drink the mixture throughout the day.
- Drink 8 ounces of water and continue to drink water throughout the day.
- Go to your health club when it is convenient. Complete your third circuit-training workout using a personal training session. You should decide at this point if you need additional personal training sessions. Personal training is expensive; however, using correct form during your strength-training sessions is critical. Make your decision accordingly.

Highlights from My Day 8:

259.5 POUNDS! I was officially in the 250s. Technically my weight loss was 11.5 pounds. Mentally, I had traveled from the 270s to the 250s. I drank a few servings of my cleanse mixture throughout the morning and went to the gym at 1 PM. Inspired that I had reached the 250s, I completed a full circuit-training workout and a 30-minute cardio session on the stationary bike. I found the stationary bike to be more difficult than the treadmill and the elliptical machine. I decided to set a goal of being able to complete a one-hour medium-intensity stationary bike cardio-session within a month. I was clearly committed not just to weight loss but also to exercise. I was not only losing weight, my mental outlook toward health and fitness had clearly changed— only eight days into my program.

DAY 9

- Wake up, use the bathroom, and weigh yourself.
- Prepare your Master Cleanse Mixture. Drink your first serving and continue to drink the mixture throughout the day.
- Drink 8 ounces of water and continue to drink water throughout the day.
- Go to your health club when it is convenient. Using the knowledge you acquired from your third personal training session, complete another circuit-training workout on your own.
- Drink a serving of Traditional Medicinals Smooth Move Tea before bed.

Highlights from My Day 9:

I woke up and weighed myself—257.5 pounds. Although I felt great, my energy levels were noticeably low. I quickly drank two servings of the Master Cleanse Mixture and went to the gym. I used the limited amount of energy I had to complete a low-intensity strength-training session. I did not do any cardio exercise because I knew I did not have the energy for it. This was not discouraging for me.

I realized for the first time that I was constantly aware of exactly how my body was feeling—more than I ever had been before. Throughout each day I was able to feel incidental changes in my energy levels. I could physically feel the difference between being hungry and being thirsty. This spoke volumes about how much healthier I had become in a very short amount of time.

DAY 10

- Wake up, use the bathroom, and weigh yourself.
- Prepare your Master Cleanse Mixture. Drink your first serving and continue to drink the mixture throughout the day.
- Drink 8 ounces of water and continue to drink water throughout the day.
- Take the day off from going to your health club.

Assuming you are on the Master Cleanse, you have to make another decision. Per the original Master Cleanse book by Stanley Burroughs, you have the option of making Day 10 your last day on the cleanse. Should you choose to do this, skip to Day 15 and follow the emerging from the cleanse instructions.

Should you choose to remain on the Master Cleanse for two weeks like I did, continue to follow the guide. You should feel pretty fantastic about what you have accomplished so far! I hope you have received lots of praise from those who are following your progress.

Highlights from My Day 10:
I never considered making Day 10 my last day. I was committed to the Master Cleanse for two weeks. My weight had dropped to 256 pounds—down 15 pounds. My skin looked great, my body felt great, and I was not about to stray from my original plan. I did not miss my former diet. The thought of it began to disgust me. I did take the day off from going to the gym.

DAY 11

- Wake up, use the bathroom, and weigh yourself.
- Prepare your Master Cleanse Mixture. Drink your first serving and continue to drink the mixture throughout the day.
- Drink 8 ounces of water and continue to drink water throughout the day.
- Go to your health club when it is convenient. Depending on what your energy levels are, engage in any light form of circuit-training or cardiovascular exercise.
- Drink a serving of Traditional Medicinals Smooth Move Tea before bed.

Highlights from My Day 11:

I woke up on Day 11 weighing 253.5 pounds—down another 2.5 pounds. My energy levels were great. I drank two servings of the Master Cleanse Mixture and went to the gym early in the morning. I listened to my iTunes and completed an enjoyable one-hour medium-intensity cardio workout on the elliptical machine. Because I still had plenty of energy after my cardio workout, I completed a light strength-training session.

DAY 12

- Wake up, use the bathroom, and weigh yourself.
- Prepare your Master Cleanse Mixture. Drink your first serving and continue to drink the mixture throughout the day.
- Drink 8 ounces of water and continue to drink water throughout the day.
- If you have the energy, go to your health club when it is convenient. Engage in any light form of cardiovascular exercise.

Highlights from My Day 12:

I woke up and saw that my weight had dropped to 252.5 pounds. Day 12 was a low-energy day for me. I decided to take the day off from working out. Knowing my cleanse would end in two days, I started reading article after article online about nutrition.

> **IMPORTANT:** Exercise is optional and not required during the next five days if you are using the Master Cleanse for two weeks. You will complete the Master Cleanse on Day 14, spend the following three days coming off of the cleanse, and transition into your new permanent healthy-eating program.

DAY 13

- Wake up, use the bathroom, and weigh yourself.
- Prepare your Master Cleanse Mixture. Drink your first serving and continue to drink the mixture throughout the day.
- Drink 8 ounces of water and continue to drink water throughout the day.
- Take the day off from going to the gym.
- Drink a serving of Traditional Medicinals Smooth Move Tea before bed.

Weather permitting; walk a mile outside (if you are up to it). Celebrate the fact that tomorrow will be your last day on the Master Cleanse. Think about how far you have come in such a short time.

Highlights from My Day 13:
I awakened weighing 251 pounds. Although my energy levels were low, I otherwise felt great. I drank three servings of the Master Cleanse Mixture in the morning and went to the gym in the early afternoon. I decided not to attempt any cardio due to my low energy levels and opted for a strength-training workout session instead. During my second exercise in the second rotation of my strength-training circuit, my arms started cramping. I immediately stood up, smiled, walked out of the gym, and drank a serving of my Master Cleanse Mixture before driving home. I knew I would not resume my exercise program until I started eating again.

I was not discouraged or upset because I could not complete my strength-training session. I had lost a remarkable amount of weight in a very short period of time. I was breathing better, sleeping better, and mentally prepared to lose all of the remaining weight I needed to lose. Incredibly, the Traditional Medicinals Smooth Move Tea was still doing its job—on Day 13! Draw your own conclusions about the level of toxicity that was present in my body if I was still able to eliminate on the thirteenth day while I was on the Master Cleanse.

People were starting to become aware of my progress and were in disbelief that I had not eaten (chewed) anything for almost two weeks. Most were surprised that I was still functioning at a very high level. I was not surprised because I knew my body was receiving the nutrients it needed to sustain itself.

DAY 14

- Wake up, use the bathroom, and weigh yourself.
- Prepare your Master Cleanse Mixture. Drink your first serving and continue to drink the mixture throughout the day.
- Drink 8 ounces of water and continue to drink water throughout the day.
- Take the day off from going to the gym.
- Go to the store and buy a gallon of fresh squeezed orange juice (substitute pineapple juice if you prefer). Buy organic low or no sodium soup broths (multiple flavors). Additionally, buy enough organic fruits and vegetables to last for the next few days.
- Get ready to transition into your permanent healthy-eating program.

Highlights from My Day 14:

I woke up weighing 249 pounds—22 pounds lost in two weeks. I knew I would never weigh over 250 pounds again! I felt fantastic. Lisa was very proud of me and knew I was finally committed to living a long, healthy life. Although I was currently taking a few days off from exercise, I knew physical fitness would always be part of my life. I could not have mentally prepared myself better to continue on my weight-loss program.

DAY 15

- Wake up, use the bathroom, and weigh yourself. Document your weight. Time to ease your body off of the Master Cleanse! Think about what you have accomplished.
- Drink 8 ounces of fresh squeezed orange juice (or pineapple juice).
- Drink 8 ounces of water and continue to drink water throughout the day.
- Drink five or six 8-oz. servings of juice throughout the day.

Highlights from My Day 15:

I weighed 248 pounds on the morning of Day 15, which meant that I had lost a total of 23 pounds since I started the Master Cleanse. I had been concerned about only consuming orange juice (and water, of course) for the entire day. It was surprisingly much easier than I thought it would be. Completing two weeks on the Master Cleanse became quite the story in my immediate circle of close friends and family. No one (including me) could imagine what was yet to come.

DAY 16

- Wake up, use the bathroom, and weigh yourself.
- Drink a glass of fresh squeezed orange juice or pineapple juice.
- Drink 8 ounces of water and continue to drink water throughout the day.
- Enjoy a warm cup of organic soup. Drink up to five servings of soup throughout the day.
- Go to the store or farmers market and buy more organic fruits and vegetables. Make sure you buy enough to last for a few days.

Highlights from My Day 16:

Because I was only eating soup on Day 16, I enjoyed a bowl of organic lemon grass soup for breakfast. I know this must sound bizarre; however, Day 16 would be the day I adopted the idea that as long as I was eating wholesome, unprocessed or minimally processed food, I could eat anything that appealed to me at any time of the day. I would no longer limit myself to eating breakfast-specific meals in the morning, lunch-specific meals in the afternoon, and dinner-specific meals in the evening. I ate single-cup bowls of organic lemon grass soup and organic mushroom soup on Day 16, consuming a total of five bowls. I looked forward to chewing food on Day 17.

DAY 17

- Wake up, use the bathroom, and weigh yourself.
- Drink 8 ounces of water and continue to drink water throughout the day.
- This is your last day to ease off of the Master Cleanse. Go to your chosen grocery store, healthy café, and restaurant and buy enough healthy convenience foods to last for two or three days. Enjoy the experience—you are about to begin your permanent healthy eating program. When you get back home chop vegetables, separate chicken, cut up fruit, and place your convenience foods in sealable storage containers in your refrigerator.

Breakfast:
Enjoy a cup of fresh organic strawberries mixed with raspberries. Chew the fruit thoroughly.

Approximately Three Hours Later:
Enjoy a warm cup of soup with vegetables. Chew the vegetables thoroughly.

Approximately Three Hours Later:
Enjoy another warm cup of soup with vegetables. Chew the vegetables thoroughly.

Approximately Three Hours Later:
Eat another cup of fruit. Chew the fruit thoroughly.

Approximately Three Hours Later:
Enjoy a cup of soup with vegetables. Chew the vegetables thoroughly.

Highlights from My Day 17:
I woke up weighing 245 pounds. I felt like a new person. The menu you see above for Day 17 is what I ate on my own Day 17. I looked forward to Day 18 when I would be able to start my healthy-eating program and resume my exercise program.

DAY 18

Congratulations, you are chewing food again! You will notice that the food consumption I recommend each day is matched with proposed exercise requirements. You should now be accustomed to drinking substantial amounts of water. Drinking substantial amounts of water and eating nutrient-dense food every day will make it easy for your body to tell you when you are full. You should not have the desire to overeat. Eat until you feel satiated and know that you can eat again whenever you are hungry. Immediately start eating small servings of nutrient-dense food multiple times each day.

Today you begin your permanent healthy-eating program and resume your workout program! Eat at least two times today before exercising. All food recommendations listed below are from my own Healthy and Convenient Food List. The food choices I am recommending for the next three days are from my own Healthy and Convenient Food List. Feel free to incorporate your own healthy food selections based on your personal preferences and add them to the items from my Healthy and Convenient Food List.

- Wake up, use the bathroom, and weigh yourself.
- Drink 8 ounces of water and continue to drink water throughout the day.

Exercise Requirement for the Day:
Go to your health club when it is convenient.

Strength training: Complete a strength-training workout.

Cardio: Complete a 30-minute low-intensity cardio session.

Breakfast
Eat a half cup of high protein plain Greek yogurt—one that is not made with sweeteners or other additives. Mix in a small handful of organic granola, a small handful of organic trail mix, and a few organic blueberries. Add organic Grade B dark amber maple syrup and organic sugar to taste.

Approximately Three Hours Later:
Eat two hard-boiled eggs (or egg whites).

Approximately Two Hours Later:
Eat a handful of organic trail mix.

Approximately Three Hours Later:
Eat a healthy turkey sandwich on organic whole grain bread with organic canola mayonnaise, organic tomato, organic onion, organic basil, and a few organic blue corn chips.

Approximately Three Hours Later:
Heat up and eat a small serving of all natural cooked chicken and sliced organic grilled vegetables from storage containers in your refrigerator.

Highlights from My Day 18:
I completed a full strength-training workout and a 30-minute low-intensity cardio session on the elliptical machine. I was excited to eat healthy food and start exercising again. I ate until I was full, did not overeat, and had no desire to consume any highly processed foods. As usual, I drank a gallon of water throughout the day.

> **IMPORTANT**: This is the first time you will be applying the healthy eating principles described in this book to your own diet. Now is a great time to become an expert food purchaser. READ LABELS to ensure that you are buying nutrient-dense food. PLAN AHEAD so that you always have healthy meals readily available.

DAY 19

- Wake up, use the bathroom, and weigh yourself.
- Drink eight ounces of water and continue to drink water throughout the day.

Exercise Requirement for the Day:
Cardio: Complete one hour of easy cardio exercise. You may combine 30 minutes of two different types of cardio (i.e. stationary bike and treadmill). Alternatively, exercise outside for an hour by taking a fast-paced walk or slow run.

Enjoy a small dessert 15 minutes prior to your cardio session.

Breakfast:
Toast two Nature's Path Organic Flax Plus Waffles. Enjoy with a teaspoon of organic butter or Earth Balance natural buttery spread, and a side of organic Grade B dark amber maple syrup. Alternatively, eat your waffles with a topping of high-protein yogurt mixed with berries, a little organic sugar, and organic trail mix. Enjoy an 8-oz. glass of fresh squeezed orange, pineapple, or grapefruit juice.

Approximately Three Hours Later:
Eat a small turkey sandwich with organic blue corn chips.

Approximately Two Hours Later:
Eat a 4-oz. serving of organic trail mix.

Approximately Three Hours Later:
Eat a 6-oz. serving of broccoli burst salad.

Approximately Three Hours Later:
Eat a small serving of a healthfully prepared takeout dish from one of your chosen restaurants.

Highlights from My Day 19:
I accomplished the goal I had set for myself on Day 8 and completed a one-hour medium-intensity cardio session on the stationary bike. This was only the beginning of my achievements related to exercise that I would accomplish in 2011. As usual, I drank a gallon of water throughout the day.

DAY 20

- Wake up, use the bathroom, and weigh yourself.
- Drink 8 ounces of water and continue to drink water throughout the day.

Exercise Requirement for the Day:
Go to your health club when it is convenient.

Strength training: Complete a strength-training workout.
Cardio: Complete a 30-minute medium-intensity cardio workout.
This is a big exercise day. You need to make sure to eat accordingly. Now that you understand how to make healthy eating flexible and convenient, you can easily match your food consumption with your planned exercise for each day. You will notice that I have recommended that you eat heartily today. Enjoy!

Breakfast:
Eat four hard boiled eggs (or egg whites) and a 5-oz. serving of high protein yogurt. Mix in a small handful of organic granola, a small handful of organic trail mix, and a few berries. Add organic Grade B dark amber maple syrup or organic sugar to taste.

Approximately Three Hours Later:
Eat a cup of quinoa salad.

Approximately Two Hours Later:
Eat four ounces of organic trail mix.

Approximately Three Hours Later:
Eat a whole sliced organic avocado topped with chopped organic red onions and a pinch of organic sea salt. Drizzle a little organic olive oil on top. Enjoy this healthy snack with some organic blue corn chips.

Approximately Three Hours Later:
Prepare a quick stir fry using the meat and vegetables you have conveniently stored in your refrigerator. Enjoy a few bites of organic ice cream, you deserve it!

Highlights from My Day 20:
I woke up and weighed myself—243 pounds! I was so excited. I could not believe I had lost almost 30 pounds. I killed it at the gym on Day 20. I completed a full strength-training session and another one-hour medium-intensity workout on the seated stationary bike—proving that what I accomplished the day before was not a fluke. During the evening of Day 20 I soaked in an Epsom salt bath and slept soundly for eight hours. I highly recommend taking Epsom salt baths on strenuous exercise days.

DAY 21

- Wake up, use the bathroom, and weigh yourself.
- Drink 8 ounces of water and continue to drink water throughout the day.

Assuming you followed my recommendation and started your final weight loss on a Monday morning, Day 21 falls on a Sunday. Now that you are chewing food again, Sunday should to be the start of the first full week that you are able to complete the requirements included in the 5-95 Weight-Loss Exercise Program.

Exercise Requirement for the Day:
You have options! If you followed my recommended workouts for the last three days, feel free to take the day off—you have all week to fulfill your exercise requirements. Should you choose to take the day off from strenuous exercise, engage in a relaxing, enjoyable physical activity. Your activity might include a round of golf, a hike to a beautiful location, or a long walk on a beach.

Should you choose not to take the day off from exercise, complete a one-hour medium-intensity cardio session—leaving four hours of cardio to be completed during the remainder of the week to fulfill your cardio requirement on the 5-95 Weight-Loss Exercise Program.

Breakfast:
Go to a healthy café or restaurant that serves wholesome, healthfully prepared food. Enjoy a latte' made with organic coffee beans and organic non-fat milk. Alternatively, enjoy a serving of organic green tea. Eat part of an organic egg white omelet filled with organic cheese and organic vegetables. Enjoy with a side of salsa. Eat a piece of whole grain toast. Take the remainder of the omelet you could not finish to go and enjoy it later as a full meal or as a side dish with another meal.

Approximately Three Hours Later:
Eat ¾ of a cup of broccoli burst salad.

Approximately Three Hours Later:
Drink a healthy shake made with Dream Protein Powder.

Approximately Two Hours Later:
Eat a handful of trail mix.

Approximately Three Hours Later:
Heat up chicken and vegetables. Enjoy with a small side of organic sweet potato fries. Enjoy a couple glasses of wine with dinner and celebrate your commitment to your final weight loss.

Highlights from My Day 21:
I woke up and was sore from my workouts on Day 20. I knew I would not be doing any strength training at the gym. I ate breakfast and went to the driving range at the golf course instead. I had lost almost 30 pounds in three weeks and needed to work on my terrible golf swing. I developed a new and unfamiliar golf swing due to my weight loss—my old golf swing was not anything to write home about so it did not make that much of a difference to me. One of the unfortunate aspects of my new swing was that my club head was hitting the ground before making contact with the golf ball. I was no longer taking as wide a swing as I had been before I started losing weight because I did not have as much mass to swing around. My patient golf instructor informed me that since I did not have as much mass on my body to swing around, I was releasing my club head too early on the down swing and my swing path had become too steep. I didn't care. My golf game was the only aspect of my life that was suffering as a result of my weight loss. Everything else was an enormous upgrade. I spent two hours shanking balls, left the golf course, and went to the gym. I completed a one-hour cardio session on the elliptical machine, drove home, and enjoyed a couple of glasses of wine with Lisa at dinner. I was celebrating! I knew I was going to lose the remainder of my weight and never be overweight again.

Summary

The guidelines in this chapter should give you a good idea of what to look forward to during your first three weeks of weight loss. I saw and felt the results of being on my weight-loss program for only three weeks and knew I would lose the remaining weight I needed to lose permanently and never be overweight again.

Establishing healthy living patterns such as eating small amounts of food throughout the day, drinking water consistently throughout the day, and committing to a weekly exercise program will become routine for you—just as your former unhealthy living patterns became routine.

I could not have imagined all of the things that would become possible in my world when I started losing weight on my self-designed weight-loss program. When you read Chapter 10, you should become inspired and start dreaming about what will become possible in your world when you lose your weight!

Enjoy your final weight loss—follow my program and your results will be fantastic!

Chapter NINE

WEIGHT MAINTENANCE

Unfortunately, there are numerous gimmicky weight loss programs that only provide a temporary solution. When these gimmicky programs (shake replacements for meals every day, starvation diets, no-carb diets, etc.) are discontinued, the weight comes right back on and more is often added. This scenario is so commonplace that our society has become resigned to it. Before my own final weight loss, engaging in gimmicky weight-loss programs and regaining all of my weight back and adding more had been my modus operandi for 27 years.

The Mental Aspect of Weight Maintenance

Once you have determined in your own mind that being overweight or obese has become unbearable, the changes you make in your life should be permanent ones so that you will never be overweight again. Put another way, you must adopt new living habits that include a different way of approaching diet and exercise that will accommodate your weight loss permanently. When I hear people tell me that despite their intense desire to lose weight, they don't have enough time or money to incorporate a healthy way of living into their life on a permanent basis, the only thought that enters my mind is "it is not your time, that is the problem."

Please know that "it is not your time" does not mean that you are a failure or a loser. It simply means that you have not made the mental commitment to live your life differently in order to lose weight and maintain a healthy weight for the rest of your life.

Knowing That You Will Never Be Overweight Again

You know you will never be overweight again when you have mentally "flipped the switch," and unhealthy patterns in your previous lifestyle no longer appeal to you. You have accepted the fact that in the grand scheme of things, nothing is more important than your health. Here are some examples of conscious health decisions that you should make if you are committed to never being overweight again:

You no longer consider exercise to be optional. Despite your personal obligations and challenges, you have found a way to incorporate a meaningful, consistent exercise program into your life every week.

You have concluded that although highly processed, nutrient-poor foods are convenient, you will avoid them whenever possible and not consider it an indulgence to eat them. You know that no amount of exercise will make up for a poor diet, and it is not worth it from a health perspective to choose to eat unhealthy. You are more than willing to subject yourself to a minimal amount of inconvenience at various times (i.e., while traveling) to eat healthy food rather than unhealthy food.

You know that in order to maintain a healthy weight you should never force yourself to eat less food or spend any time during the day being hungry. You should eat nutrient-dense foods often and in substantial enough quantities to feel satisfied without ever feeling stuffed.

You drink considerable amounts of water throughout each day and easily avoid all types of soda and highly processed sugary fruit drinks that contain little to no real fruit juice. Drinking substantial amounts of water has become a habit for you. You no longer have a desire to consume full-sugar soda, diet soda, or highly processed sugary fruit drinks. You readily acknowledge that drinking nutrient-poor beverages is as bad for you as eating nutrient-poor food and you are no longer tempted to purchase these well-marketed, commercially sold products.

The Bottom Line on Weight Maintenance

The patterns I have listed above are examples of how a person chooses to live if he or she never wants to be overweight or obese again. These are permanent lifestyle changes, not temporary changes. One should never lose weight for a specific event such as a party, wedding, or weight-loss contest as this is an invitation to fail at weight maintenance on a permanent basis.

Taking Full Advantage of Your Permanent Weight Loss and Future Weight Maintenance

Once you have lost a substantial amount of weight on a sustainable weight-loss program and have established healthy living patterns on a permanent basis, a whole new world will open up for you. You will give yourself the opportunity to participate in activities, accomplish personal goals, and live dreams that would have never been possible had you not decided to take your fate in your own hands. Turn the page and read what became possible for me. While you are reading about what became possible for me, think about your own dreams and aspirations. Enjoy what will become possible in your world as you continue to live your life as someone who no longer has a weight problem.

Chapter TEN

WHAT BECOMES POSSIBLE

A couple of weeks into July 2011, I was talking with a friend of mine who has always been health conscious and very fit. I told her that I had finally decided to commit to a healthy lifestyle and enthusiastically shared that I had lost 42 pounds in less than three months. When she asked how I had done it, I described my self-designed weight-loss program including the 5-95 Weight-Loss Exercise Program.

She lives in Las Vegas and suggested that I start training and try to run the Zappos.com Las Vegas Rock and Roll Half Marathon with her on December 4, 2011. Although running a half-marathon sounded like it would be very personally rewarding, the only cardio exercise I was doing that resembled running was medium-paced walking on a treadmill at my gym. Our phone call ended with my deciding to try to run a mile the following day.

I arrived at my gym the next morning and easily ran a 12.5-minute mile. It was not as difficult as I imagined it would be. The next day I ran two miles. During the next three weeks, two miles became three miles and three miles became five miles (all on a treadmill). I continued to follow my 5-95 Weight-Loss Exercise Program requirements. Running became a cardio substitution within my 5-95 Program for the stationary bike and elliptical machine. I was not adding more time to my cardio regimen each week; I was simply using a different type of cardio exercise (this illustrates how you can easily modify my 5-95 Weight-Loss Exercise Program to meet different workout goals).

I was not fully committed to running the half-marathon in Las Vegas; however, it was starting to seem like more of a possibility. I had been running for three weeks and was already able to run five miles on a treadmill. My weight continued to come off. The more weight I lost, the more confident I became. I reached the three month anniversary of starting my weight-loss program and had already lost more than 50 pounds. I flew to Orlando, Florida to attend a convention. Flying from Eugene to Orlando gave me a lot of downtime to mull over the idea of running a half-marathon.

I was enjoying a glass of wine on my return flight and pulled up the Zappos.com Las Vegas Marathon website. The event website was awesome—it showcased running down the Las Vegas Strip at night with bands playing at various locations along the course. Given that the event was at the beginning of December, I would have just over four months to train. I could only imagine how much lighter I would be in four months.

Running a half-marathon is more than admirable, but why run a half-marathon when the wine and my own sense of accomplishment told me I could run a full marathon? The only aspect of running this particular marathon that seemed troubling to me was that it had a 4.5-hour finishing time limit. I figured this was an approximate time limit and assumed that if I trained properly, I would be able to do it—what in the hell did I know? I whipped out my credit card, registered online, and that was it, I was officially registered to run a full marathon!

When Lisa picked me up at the airport in Eugene, I gave her the exciting news. I told her all about the website, the bands, running on the Las Vegas Strip at night, the crowds, and how excited I was.

Ever the practical one, Lisa said, "Let me get this straight. You are telling me you are going to run a full marathon? You have never run anything before—what about your ankle?"

I had suffered a left ankle injury a few years earlier. We were at the

Oregon coast with friends. I tried to carry a large box down some stairs while wearing golf shoes. My soft spikes dug into the rug on the stairs and all 270+ pounds of me tumbled down the stairs. Although I didn't break any bones, I did sustain soft tissue injuries around my left ankle and did not complete the appropriate amount of physical therapy to heal myself. My left ankle was a concern; however, it did not bother me nearly as much as it had when I had been 50 pounds heavier.

Lisa and I agreed (Lisa insisted and I agreed) that I have a consultation with the physical therapy clinic she was using to rehabilitate her shoulder. Cooperative Performance and Rehabilitation in Eugene offers a bio-mechanical assessment program called The RunWell Program, created by Robert Wayner, PT. This sport-specific performance training program is designed to meet the needs of runners regardless of age, experience, or level of competition.

Given the fact that I was middle aged, had no experience running, and had not yet established a level of competition, the RunWell Program was perfect for me. During my first meeting with Robert, I explained I had lost <u>54 pounds</u> in just over three months and had signed up to run in the Las Vegas Marathon on December 4. Being an experienced runner and athlete himself, Robert assured me that he could help me. I asked Robert if he created marathon programs for first-time runners. He told me that he did not design training programs for people but would be happy to refer me to a running coach who could strategize a training program for me. He generously offered to arrange an appointment where we could all meet during my second RunWell Program Appointment. During my second appointment, Robert would be doing a full biomechanical assessment of my strength and flexibility, and assessing my injuries.

The running coach Robert referred me to was Cathie Twomey Bellamy. Cathie and I exchanged a casual email and agreed to meet at my second RunWell appointment. I found out later that she and Robert were also exchanging emails about me. Cathie had serious issues with the fact that I was planning to run a marathon and did not have any running experience other than running a few miles on the treadmill. She initially told Robert to tell me to go run a 5K (translation: I will not indulge this wine-induced pipe dream. Please convince this person that he needs to run shorter distance races first before attempting a marathon). Robert told her that I was hell-bent on running a marathon before the end of the year. As a favor to him, Cathie agreed to show up to my appointment and talk some sense into me.

When Cathie arrived at Cooperative Performance and Rehabilitation, my second RunWell Appointment was already underway. I was lying on the examination table and Robert was assessing my strength and flexibility (i.e., my lack of strength and flexibility). Lisa was with me because she wanted to meet Cathie and see my biomechanical assessment first hand. Needless to say, Lisa also had some serious concerns about my marathon plans. Cathie had barely introduced herself to us when she turned to me and asked me why I wanted to run a marathon.

I answered with the following: "I have lost 57 pounds since April 25, 2011. I feel like I can accomplish anything at this point, including running a full marathon."

Cathie looked at Lisa and said, "57 pounds in just over three months? How is this possible?" Lisa pulled out her iPad and started showing Cathie pre-weight-loss pictures of me from early 2011. Cathie was duly impressed and suggested a half-marathon instead of the 5K she had in mind when she first arrived. The miracle of weight-loss confidence was officially spreading beyond the wine from my return plane flight from Orlando.

My response to Cathie's suggestion that I run a half-marathon: "If I am going to do this, I am going to do the whole damn thing."

I can only imagine how insane that must have sounded to someone with Cathie's background and expertise (I was unaware of Cathie's background as a legendary world class runner). Following my outrageous declaration, Robert put me on the treadmill in his office and had me run at a 5-mile per hour pace. Cathie, Robert, and Lisa stood about twelve feet behind the treadmill and discussed my running stride. Cathie was hoping that I would have a terrible foot plant so she could immediately tell me that training for a marathon was out of the question—she desperately wanted to tell me to run a 5K and be done with this once and for all. Apparently, I had a great foot plant and a pretty decent running stride (not attributable to anything other than luck). After watching me run on the treadmill, Cathie looked at Robert and said, "What have you gotten me into?" She agreed to put a training program together for me and left.

That was August 16, 2011. Now I had a running coach. I had no idea at the time what a "foot plant" was. As far as I was concerned, running was putting one foot in front of the other and moving more quickly than walking. I was clueless.

I never asked Cathie for a list of her qualifications. She entered the room with a swagger, looked like a runner, and had been recommended by Robert Wayner for whom I already had a tremendous amount of respect. That was more than enough for me. The fact that I had never heard of Cathie shows that I was completely out of my league.

Based on the preliminary information Robert gave to Cathie from my RunWell biomechanical assessment, she decided that my first long run would be six miles. My assessment revealed that I needed to greatly increase my strength and flexibility if I was to have a prayer of completing a full marathon. The RunWell Program book Robert prepared for me provided me with stretching exercises that would increase my overall strength and flexibility. He also gave me exercises to rehab my left ankle. It has truly been a privilege for me to have the opportunity to work with Robert.

Cathie informed me that my six-mile run and all future "long training runs" would be completed outside on pavement. My six-mile run was to be completed by Monday August 29 (I would be out of town during the third week in August). Cathie and I would reconnect on Tuesday, August 30, and plan the details of my next long-run based on how I felt after running six miles.

Running a marathon was something I used to dream about in fantasy weight-loss dreams. I had never trained for one. I used to imagine what it would be like to be in the kind of shape one would need to be in to run a marathon—and then I would gain more weight. Things were different this time! I had already lost more weight than I ever had in other weight-loss attempts and I had permanently changed my life. Although I was in fantastic shape from a cardio fitness perspective, I was still light years away from being physically prepared to run a marathon—I just didn't know it.

Lisa and I were enjoying wine with friends one evening prior to my first outdoor long training run when she proudly and enthusiastically let the cat out of the bag and told everyone that I was going to run a full marathon in December. "Jase" and "marathon" were now officially being used in the same sentence by a number of people who knew me (even if the sentence was "Jase is an idiot if he thinks he is going to run a full marathon in less than four months"). I continued to run on the treadmill until August 29. The reason I continued to run on the treadmill and not on the pavement until I attempted my six mile outdoor long-run was because I did not want the dream to die. What if running on a paved road was much more difficult than a treadmill? What if my ankle was in too much pain and I could not complete a six mile run on pavement?

Marathon Training Runs, Mistakes, and Milestones
Monday, August 29, 2011
I mapped out my six-mile run on a one-mile paved road down the hill from our house. My six-mile run would be in the books if I could run three round trip laps. Monday evening I drove down the hill, parked next to the paved road, put in my ear buds, turned on my iPod, and ran six miles. Running on a paved road was much different from running

on a treadmill; however, it was not as difficult as I had imagined. Running outside was a hell of a lot more interesting than running indoors. Looking at trees, mountains, and other aspects of nature while running and listening to music was something I knew I would enjoy during my future outdoor training runs. I was so relieved to have my first pavement run behind me. I emailed Cathie and informed her that my six-mile long run had gone well and was looking forward to her next instruction—sort of.

Sunday, September 4, 2011

Cathie informed me earlier in the week that I would be running eight miles on Sunday, September 4. I would start the run at Alton Baker Park in Eugene. Alton Baker Park is near Autzen Stadium (where the University of Oregon Ducks play football) and is located near a 12-mile running/bike trail called the Ruth Bascom Riverbank Trail System. The trails flank both sides of the Willamette River. I easily ran eight miles. The paths were clearly marked and I was able to run along the north bank trail, cross over the Greenway Bike Bridge, run down the south bank trail, and backtrack to my car. My average mile pace was approximately 11 minutes and 15 seconds. I emailed Cathie and informed her that I had run eight miles successfully without incident but would like to meet with her in person for a strategy talk because I had a concern about the specific marathon that I had chosen to run. She agreed to meet me for coffee in Eugene on Tuesday.

Following my eight-mile run, I contacted the Zappos.com Las Vegas Rock and Roll Marathon representative and inquired about their required time limit of 4.5 hours. Was this a suggested time limit? How was this enforced? What happens if I don't finish in 4.5 hours?

The answers to these questions by the very nice gentleman on the other end of the phone went something like this, "The time limit is 4.5 hours firm. If you are not at the half-way mark in two hours and 15 minutes we will stop you, put you on a bus, and drive you to the finish area—your marathon will be over."

I must admit that in my chardonnay-infused plane flight from Orlando to Eugene, riding on the loser bus to the finish line because I could not get to the half-way point in two hours and 15 minutes was not part of my grand plan. My "curiosity question" to Cathie, my sympathetic running coach, the following day would be, "Do we think that I will be able to improve my current 11:15 average mile running pace over 8 miles to a 10:30 average mile running pace over, say…26.2 miles in the next three months?" Poor woman…what in the hell did she ever do to deserve this?

Cathie Twomey Bellamy, a former world class runner turned running/track coach in Eugene (otherwise known as Track Town USA), agrees to meet with former 271-pound treadmill alum Jase Simmons for a marathon strategy session. Could this possibly get more absurd? Yes, much more absurd.

After talking with the representative in Las Vegas, I decided to establish a back-up plan in case we (Cathie) decided that I would not be able to shave 45 seconds off of my average mile. I decided to come to our meeting prepared so I searched for another marathon to run in December, 2011. There was no chance that I was not going to attempt a marathon in 2011. Running a marathon in the same calendar year that my miraculous weight loss and lifestyle transformation was taking place had become very important to me.

I originally decided that I was going to travel all the way to the opposite side of the world from being overweight. Running a marathon would be the ultimate confirmation of my complete lifestyle change. I typed "2011 marathon schedule" into the Google search engine and found a list of all marathons taking place in 2011. I immediately scrolled down to the month of December. I knew I needed time to train (much more time than I was giving myself). The Honolulu Marathon was the week after the Zappos.com Las Vegas Marathon. I logged into the Honolulu Marathon website and learned that the Honolulu Marathon did not have a finishing time limit. Flying to Honolulu from Oregon is easy. Lisa and I could fly on a direct 4.5-hour flight from Portland. We would arrive on December 9, I would run (attempt to run) the marathon on Sunday, December 11 and return home the next day. I decided I would run the Honolulu Marathon if Cathie advised against trying to train for a 4:30:00 time limit in Las Vegas—problem solved.

Tuesday, September 6, 2011 Marathon Strategy Conversation

Cathie showed up early for our meeting and was waiting for me when I arrived. I have no idea what she saw in me. She knew that I did not have a clue about what the hell I was getting myself into. I voiced my concerns about the required time limit to complete the marathon in Vegas. She diplomatically informed me that my 11:15 average mile pace running eight miles was not going to improve to a 10:30 average mile pace running 26.2 miles in the next three months. Even though I knew almost nothing about running, I knew she would say that.

Cathie immediately recommended that I not set myself up for failure when the goal was simply to finish a marathon. She had a back-up plan already in place. She wanted me to run the Napa Valley Marathon, which would take place in March 2012. Cathie's reasoning was very sound. The Napa Valley Marathon had a six-hour time limit and she would have time to properly prepare me to be a first-time marathoner. I told her that I also had a back-up plan. Grimacing, she asked me what my plan was. I told her that if I could not run the marathon in Las Vegas on December 4, I would run the Honolulu Marathon the following week on December 11. I explained that the Honolulu Marathon had no maximum time limit and shared with her that it had become very important to me to run a marathon in the same calendar year that I was permanently losing my excess weight and changing my life forever. She quickly warned me about the heat and humidity involved with running a marathon in Honolulu. Once again, sound advice fell on deaf ears.

For whatever reason (the humor aspect was in play here for sure), Cathie agreed to craft an alternate program for me to run the Honolulu Marathon. Immediately after our meeting, I registered for the Honolulu Marathon, booked plane flights for Lisa and me, and prepaid our hotel room. There was no turning back now. I would be running in the Honolulu Marathon on December 11. Needless to say, Lisa was not opposed to the change in venue.

Sunday, September 11, 2011

The treadmill king had graduated from running on exercise equipment to completing two long-runs on pavement. Today I would run nine miles. Similar to my eight-mile training run, my nine-mile run was an accomplishment but otherwise uneventful. It took me three days to recover from my nine-mile run (sore ankles, knees, hips, and back) instead of the one-day recovery I experienced following my eight-mile run. This could only be attributed to the fact that I received a massage immediately following my eight-mile run. Lesson learned—following each long-distance run, regardless of what town I am in, I decided I would get a post-run recovery massage.

Cathie had me on a running schedule that called for a long-run each weekend with a couple of three- or four-mile "maintenance runs" during the week (usually on Tuesday and Thursday). My weekly marathon training commitments were incorporated into my 5-95 Weight-Loss Exercise Program requirements. I committed to an hour of cross-training on a stationary bike or elliptical machine two days a week in addition to strength training three days a week. Recovering quickly from my weekend distance runs was critical. I did not have the luxury of being sore for four days following a long-run on the weekend.

Two more critical aspects of the marathon training puzzle were also put in place following my nine-mile run. I decided to try to incorporate "goo packs" (Energy Gel Packs) into my marathon training diet. A goo pack is runner speak for a small pack of gel that contains a high concentration of sodium, potassium, carbs, sugar, and caffeine. In addition to providing energy for extended cardio sessions, the primary function of a goo pack is to provide an immediate source of electrolytes to help avoid cramping. I have suffered from leg cramps and muscle spasms my entire life—they come on at a moment's notice and are extremely painful. The Power Bar Energy Gel Pack would eventually become my goo pack of choice. Most people think goo (energy gel) tastes terrible; however, the Power Bar Goo Pack tasted fine to me once I finally tried it—more on this later.

I also purchased a Garmin sports watch to track my weekend long-runs. My Garmin would prove to be a fantastic way to analyze all aspects of my long-runs including distance, route, time splits, elevation change, and calories burned. Following each long-run, I would connect the Garmin to my computer, download the information from my run, and email the file to Cathie. The information provided by the Garmin would make it possible for her to analyze most of the critical information from my run (and also would prove that I actually ran the required distance).

Saturday, September 17, 2011
Per Cathie's instruction, it was time to hit double digits on my long runs. I would be running 11 miles on September 17, 2011—a personal distance record. It was officially time for me to showcase what an inexperienced runner I was. When long distance runs hit double digits, it becomes very important to be able to readily access goo packs, snacks, and water during the run. There are two ways to do this—stash them at various points along the planned running route prior to the long-run or carry them in a pack on your person while running. I became a stasher because I did not want to put any extra weight on my body while running.

During the morning before my 11-mile run, I stashed my goods at a location where I thought the half-way distance of my run would be. Unfortunately, I got lost before the half-way point—never finding the goo packs, water, and snacks I stashed prior to the run. This was the first time (it happened more times than I care to admit) I had gotten lost on a long run. Fortunately, I was wearing my Garmin watch. Even though I was lost, I was still able to track my distance. Once I located a familiar place on my running route, I was able to take a more direct path back to my car. If I had tried to follow the rest of the original planned route, I probably would have turned an 11-mile run into a 15-mile run. I viewed the map of my Garmin data detailing my run later in the day—it clearly illustrated that I was lost and hopelessly running around in circles searching for my goo packs, water bottles, etc.

My wife and coach were very entertained by the fact that I got so lost and have teased me about it endlessly. Rather than focusing on the fact that I was a complete moron for getting lost in the first place, I chose to focus on my accomplishment. I ran 11 miles without water and goo packs and decided that I was officially in great shape!

Saturday, September 24, 2011
Yachats, Oregon would be the venue for my prescribed 10-mile run on Saturday, September 24. I decided that the route would be an easy "up and back." From where we were staying, I would run five miles north on Highway 1 to Waldport, turn around, and run south five miles back. There was only one road involved, US Highway 1—no chance of getting lost this time. There was also no chance of going without water or a goo pack during the run...yeah right. I drove to Waldport early in the morning and stashed a goo pack and water in a giant curbside planter in front of a gas station. Approximately one hour later I took off on my run. By the time I got to the planter in Waldport, someone had cleaned it out and my goo pack and water bottle were gone. I laughed about my misfortune the whole way back to the house!

Saturday, October 1, 2011
I had spent time with Cathie at her morning group workout on Thursday, September 29, and told her that I would be in Las Vegas for the weekend. I assured her that I would still be able to complete my long-run. I would run in the morning, get a recovery massage in the afternoon, and enjoy Las Vegas that evening. Cathie originally wanted me to run 13 miles. I asked her if I could run 13.1 miles since that is the distance of a half-marathon. She decided that I would run 13.2 miles. Lesson learned—no more asking for longer distances.

I must admit that I had never traveled to Las Vegas with goo packs and a Garmin sports watch in my suitcase. The venue for my 13.2-mile run would be Desert Breezes Park, which is on the corner of Desert Inn and Durango. I did not want to try to find an unfamiliar running trail or run on the streets in Las Vegas and deal with stoplights and traffic. Desert Breezes Park is very large. I decided to circle it repeatedly until my Garmin indicated that I had completed 13.2 miles.

I arrived at the park at 7:30 AM and was able to find a space in a parking lot adjacent to the sidewalk. I would run past my car each time I completed a lap around the park. This would be perfect. I could lock my goo packs and water in my car, make a slight detour, and access my nutrients. Barring my car exploding in the parking lot, I would finally get to taste the dreaded goo pack. This was fortuitous because there was no way that I would have been able to run 13.2 miles breathing the dry Las Vegas desert air without water and goo packs. The run was quite difficult given the fact that each time I circled the park, I was experiencing 546 feet of elevation change. Nonetheless, I ran 13.2 miles in 2:30:53 including all nutrient stops, water breaks, and elevation changes. This was big—I had run a half-marathon distance.

Saturday, October 8, 2011

I ran eight miles on the riverbank paths in Eugene and completed my run in 1:20:51. I clocked a great time. My running time clearly illustrated how far I had progressed in the first 40 days of marathon training. I still had a long way to go, but I was very encouraged by how far I had come. My first day of treadmill exercise on April 25 was beginning to feel like a distant memory even though it had only been five and a half months.

Saturday, October 15, 2011

The Honolulu Marathon was less than two months away. Cathie had sent me an email at the beginning of the week informing me that I would be running 16 miles on Saturday, October 15. Because of the limited amount of time she had to work with, Cathie was forced to create a "skeleton marathon training program" for me that was centered on weekend long-runs filled in with two maintenance runs (3-4 miles each) and two cross-training days each week.

October 15 would be a crucial day. I needed to prove to myself and everyone else that I could run a longer distance than a half-marathon. I had established a pattern of thinking about my weekend long runs and mentally preparing for them during the week. What would I eat the night before? What would I eat for breakfast the morning of the run? How many goo packs would I need to carry and where was I going to stash the others? Where would I stash water bottles? What route on the riverbank trails would I take?

I thought about it so much throughout each week that when Saturday finally arrived, I could not wait to go out and run. I was in fantastic mental and physical shape. Although I was eating a large amounts of food (including significant amounts of carbohydrates to fuel my exercise), I weighed less than 200 pounds. My weight had dropped below 200 pounds on September 28.

Before that date, I had not weighed less than 200 pounds since 1998. Organic avocados, Fage All Natural Low-Fat Greek Strained Yogurt, Dream Protein shakes, and organic trail mix had become primary staples of my weekly diet. I consumed whole grain pasta dishes within 24 hours of my long-runs (more on this later). Just six months earlier, I had not started my final weight loss or even conceptualized what it would be. Now I felt like an athlete! I had lost more than 70 pounds and had developed a quiet confidence that could not be shaken. I did not know how much more weight I would lose, but I knew I would never be obese again.

The only issue I encountered on my 16-mile run had to do with my Garmin. I had not properly charged it the previous evening and the battery died when I was 15.14 miles into my run. According to the Garmin, I ran 15.14 miles in 2:47:44 (averaging 11:06 per mile). In reality, I ran just over 16 miles in less than 3 hours. Mission accomplished.

Saturday, October 29, 2011

I knew this day was coming the moment I finished my 16-mile run two weeks earlier. Cathie was going ask for either 18 or 19 miles on Saturday, October 29. The email arrived at the beginning of the week with my instructions and I was correct. **She wanted me to run at least 18 but no more than 19 miles on Saturday.** I decided that I would split the difference and run 18.5 miles. I completed my 18.5-mile run in exactly 3 hours and 40 minutes.

Although my 18.5-mile run had gone well, I was concerned about being able to finish the marathon. I was convinced I had the cardio fitness to run the marathon distance. However, despite my increased flexibility, my legs were extremely sore after running 18.5 miles. My ankles, calves, quads, iliotibial bands, hips, and lower back felt like they had been used in a Boy Scout Double Figure Eight knot-tying contest. There were 43 days left until the marathon and I needed help. I had to try something new.

I contacted one of my friends, Jean Nelson, who teaches yoga in Eugene, including at the University of Oregon. I wasn't particularly interested in yoga but I knew my muscle flexibility was a joke and was willing to do anything that would help get me to the finish line in Honolulu. She agreed to give me private lessons—there was no way I was going to showcase my lack of flexibility in a class with a group of yogis (practitioners of yoga) who could scratch their left shoulder with their right pinkie toe. Similar to golf, I imagined that learning yoga would be like trying to eat soup with a knife. My instincts proved to be correct. Yoga did not come easily to me; however, Jean is a patient and thoughtful instructor and is passionate about her craft. My yoga sessions provided me with increased flexibility and were extremely beneficial during the marathon.

Although I will never be a yogi, I now understand why people practice yoga and love it. I completed eight 60-minute yoga sessions before the marathon and increased my range of motion and balance in each session. Jean taught me to focus on my breathing. I will continue to benefit from the breathing techniques I learned in my yoga sessions for the rest of my life.

Apply this Important Lesson to Weight Loss

The success of my weight-loss program gave me the confidence to dream of completing a marathon. My success gave me the courage to step outside of my comfort zone to accomplish my goals, both in losing weight and running a marathon. Just as there is a mental aspect to losing weight, there is a mental aspect to running a marathon. You must be 100% all in—if you are 99% all in, you might as well be only 1% all in.

You don't know who you are until you have seen who you can become!

Saturday, November 5, 2011

Early Saturday morning Lisa and I flew to San Francisco. Cathie had given me instructions to complete an eight-mile "short long run" since I had run 18 miles the week before. I decided I would run on Saturday afternoon before attending a function that evening. I looked forward to running in San Francisco all week. I started my run in Crissy Field and followed a series of roads and paths that led up to the Golden Gate Bridge. I ran north across the Golden Gate Bridge and back across the bridge to a trail that leads to the paths that return to Crissy Field. I continued running east to the end of Pier 39 across from Alcatraz. Running across the Golden Gate Bridge made this the most enjoyable training run I completed leading up to the marathon.

Sunday, November 6, 2011

I played golf with two of my close friends while in San Francisco on the Old Course at Half Moon Bay Golf Links. Six and a half months earlier I had been in the pro shop at that same course weighing 271 pounds with a 44-inch waist trying on a golf jacket, realizing that I was transitioning from a 2XL to a 3XL. When we played golf on November 6, I weighed 196 pounds. I wore a size L golf shirt, L jacket, and size 34 golf shorts. I was five weeks away from attempting to run a full marathon.

Conceptualize this as it Relates to Your Own Final Weight Loss
Despite the fact that I fought weight for 27 years of my life and had been clinically obese for most (if not all) of the previous 12 years, I drastically changed what my future would look like in a matter of months! You must be amenable to making changes in your own life. Do not be depressed because you allowed yourself to become overweight! Control your future health by implementing my weight-loss program. Put another way, although you may have spent years being overweight, you can change the prospects for your future in a matter of months!

Saturday, November 12, 2011
I had another short long-run this weekend; however, Cathie threw a new challenge into the mix. I would run nine miles on Saturday, November 12 and incorporate elevation changes. My instructions were to run up, down, and around Skinner Butte twice. Skinner Butte is a hill on the north edge of downtown Eugene. Running up Skinner Butte added a new dimension to my training; however, it was easily manageable and I enjoyed the view of Eugene and Autzen Stadium from the summit. I continued to run up Skinner Butte in my final training runs to prepare for running up Diamond Head during the marathon.

Cathie had informed me when I successfully completed my 18.5-mile run on October 29 that barring injury, I would be able to call myself a marathoner on December 11. I appreciated the confidence she had in me. I was 100% confident that my cardio fitness could easily take me across the finish line in Honolulu. I made no secret of this when I talked about my progress with family and friends. They were incredulous that I had enough cardio stamina to complete a full marathon. Most people who are neither runners nor athletes cannot conceptualize running 26.2 miles. My friends and family members were only starting to grasp the concept that I was no longer the 5'10", 271-pound guy they thought might not see his 50th birthday.

Finishing the marathon was now predicated on whether my feet, ankles, legs, hips, and back would be able to take the entire 26.2-mile run. I had one long training run left before the marathon—21 miles on November 19. Three weeks had lapsed since I had run an 18.5 miler. Running a 21-miler on November 19 would leave three weeks until I would be running in the Honolulu Marathon. My scheduled training runs during the next eight days were as follows:

November 19	21 miles
November 22	4 miles
November 24	4 miles
November 26	10 miles

Thirty-nine miles in eight days—time to put the first 21 behind me!

Saturday, November 19, 2011
One must be able to run 21 miles before running 26.2 miles. Similar to my 16-mile and 18.5-mile training runs, I thought about my 21-mile run all week leading up to November 19.

I had talked with a few people other than my coach who had run marathons. Everyone said that there are two segments to running a marathon: the first 20 miles and the last 6.2 miles. They all said the segment that I needed to be concerned about was the last 6.2 miles. Naturally, I was concerned about this. A 21 miler would give me a taste of what it would be like to run one mile of the last 6.2 miles.

The day before my 21-mile run, I went through all of my pre-long run routines. In addition to ingesting carbs like I was getting paid for it, I stashed plenty of goo packs and water bottles at various locations throughout my running route. I had run the entire riverbank trail system as well as the detour up and around Skinner Butte plenty of times. Additionally, I had run all of the connecting paths and knew exactly what my running route would be the following day. I wanted to put to rest any lingering doubts that I or anyone else had as to whether it would be plausible for me to run a marathon on December 11.

Saturday arrived and the weather in Eugene was exactly what one would expect in the Pacific Northwest in November—37 degrees and raining. I would be starting and finishing at the Valley River Center mall parking lot. Lisa would be waiting for me when I (hopefully) completed my run. I arrived at the parking lot at 7:30 AM. I attached my iPod to my shirt, put on my running vest, running gloves, and hat. I put in my ear buds. I flipped the switch to turn on my music and heard nothing. I peeled off my gloves and played around with my iPod for a few minutes. I knew I had charged my iPod the night before—I removed it from the charger prior to leaving that morning. I could not get my iPod to turn on—it had not charged. This was a huge problem! It was one thing to run a three- or four-mile maintenance run without music; however, running 21 miles without music was an entirely different proposition. I do not like to exercise without music. I had <u>never</u> run without music.

A decision had to be made. Do I try to run 21 miles without music and get it over with or do I postpone my run for a day and properly charge my iPod? I took five minutes, considered my options, and decided to run. I was mentally and physically ready to run. I did not want to wait a day and run on Sunday and have to answer to everyone who was aware that I was supposed to run 21 miles on Saturday. Cathie would be eagerly awaiting my Garmin report via email Saturday afternoon. If I could run 21 miles without music in the cold rain in Oregon, there would be little doubt left in my mind that I could run 26.2 miles with music in the sun in Hawaii. I started my run down the north bank trail toward the east bank trail. I immediately noticed that I was paying more attention to my surroundings because I had no music. Although the weather was ugly, the scenery was amazing. I felt very lucky to live in a town that offers so many beautiful places to run.

By the time I had completed 10 miles, my legs began to feel the distance. When I had run 18 miles, I could not wait for the run to end! I was cold, the rain had pelted me for nearly four hours, and I was down to one goo pack and a small amount of water. Once my Garmin indicated that I had run more than 18.5 miles, I was happy that I had set a new personal distance record. My euphoria was temporary because my running vest, shirt, and everything else on my person was saturated from the constant rain. I was bored as hell and ready to put this experience behind me. Once I finished my 21st and final mile of my last long training run, I had put to rest any doubt that I had what it took from a cardio perspective to run a full marathon.

I had just completed a 21-mile run in miserable conditions with no music. I arrived back at the parking lot. Lisa saw me approaching, jumped out of her car, and threw her arms around me, clearly relieved that I was physically doing well and had survived the miserable conditions. I received a fantastic massage that afternoon and my body fully recovered from the 21-mile run by the following evening.

Three Weeks until the Marathon

Cathie scaled back my running significantly during the three weeks leading up to the marathon. I ran 10 miles on November 26, nine miles on December 3, and two four-mile maintenance runs in-between. She had put together an incredible training program for me given the limited amount of time she had to work with. I could not have been more grateful to her for her time, effort, energy, and expertise. She gave me every opportunity to achieve something that I never would have dreamed possible seven months prior. I was ready to make her proud.

Chapter ELEVEN

RUNNING THE 2011 HONOLULU MARATHON

I frequently viewed the Honolulu Marathon Facebook page for updates during the month leading up to the event. Lisa and I were flying to Honolulu on Friday, two days before the marathon. I completed my last five-mile training run on Wednesday, per Cathie's instruction. Thursday, I had a check-up scheduled with my primary care physician. He had not seen me since February—two months before I began my final weight loss.

Before I saw my doctor that day, the nurse weighed me, showed me to my examination room, and took my vital signs. A short time later, my doctor walked into the examination room, said hello, and smiled as though he was familiar with me but could not place me. This was understandable because I had only seen him three times before—he works in a large practice and sees many patients every week. I had lost more than 70 pounds since the last time he had seen me. He reviewed my chart and noted my weight, heartbeat, and blood pressure numbers (194.4 pounds, 60 beats per minute, 120/70 blood pressure) and compared them with the numbers from my last office visit back in February when I weighed 268 pounds. He did a double take, looked at me, laughed, said "Holy shit," and shook my hand.

Most of the appointment was spent discussing my weight loss and how I had trained for the Honolulu Marathon. I was asking a lot of questions and wanted medical clearance to run. My doctor could tell I was nervous and finally said, "You are healthy and have obviously put in the work. Now go run." I felt so great. I had completed all the pre-marathon training runs required by my coach during the previous four months and had just received the green light from my primary care physician.

Lisa and I drove to Portland Thursday evening and spent the night at an airport hotel. We arrived at the airport the following morning, endured the long security line, and immediately went to Starbucks and waited in another long line. The long line at Starbucks could not have been more fortuitous. While we were waiting in line, we struck up a conversation with a nice lady who was flying to San Diego to see her grandchildren. Her daughter's husband was in the army and he was currently stationed in Afghanistan. When the lady asked us where we were going, Lisa told her that we were flying to Honolulu because I had lost 77 pounds and was running in the Honolulu Marathon. After congratulating me, the lady offered some words of wisdom for running a marathon. The advice she gave me would benefit me during my most critical moment of the entire marathon.

"I ran a half-marathon once", she said. "During that run, every time I thought about trying to make it to the finish line, my running became very difficult and I ran poorly. When I stayed in the moment and didn't think about crossing the finish line, I ran so much better and running immediately became much easier. When you run the Honolulu Marathon, be in the moment and don't think about the difficult parts of the course that are left for you to complete. Enjoy the experience and you will run well."

Once we received our drinks, we thanked her and wished her well, walked to the gate, and boarded our flight. Lisa started a conversation with the man seated next to us and learned that he was a civil engineer—they immediately had a lot to talk about because Lisa is also a civil engineer. He told us that he was traveling to Honolulu to run the marathon. I could not have been less surprised to hear this. He looked like a marathon runner (much more than I did, that was for sure). He went on to tell us that he was running in his second

Honolulu Marathon and lamented that he had been unable to finish the marathon in his first attempt because of a sore IT band (iliotibial band). Do I ever know about pain in the IT band!

Picture the scene. We were listening to this experienced marathon runner weighing at least 35 pounds less than me, tell us a story about how he did not finish the Honolulu Marathon in his first attempt because he sustained a painful injury in his iliotibial band. This was the last thing I needed to hear, particularly from someone who was clearly in much better shape than I was.

Thoughts began to creep into my head about my own prospects of finishing the marathon. I knew I had done everything (albeit in a limited amount of time) that I could to prepare for the marathon. I could not have had a more qualified coach prepare me with a better training program. I had never been in better shape in my life than I was at that moment. I weighed 77 pounds less than I had seven and a half months earlier. Instead of worrying about my prospects of finishing the marathon, I decided to enjoy the experience with Lisa.

We arrived in Honolulu and immediately went to the convention center to pick up my marathon packet and visit the vendor booths. I bought marathon souvenirs including a Honolulu Marathon ornament to hang on our Christmas tree knowing damn well that if I was unable to finish the marathon, the Honolulu Marathon ornament I just purchased would never make it back to Oregon, let alone hang from a branch on our Christmas tree.

When we arrived at the hotel, it was time for me to start "carbing up" for the marathon. We went to the beachside restaurant where I indulged in a grilled mahi mahi sandwich with french fries, grilled corn on the cob sautéed in butter, pepper, and parmesan cheese, and a hot fudge sundae for dessert.

Now that I sound like the biggest hypocrite on the planet based on what I have written in Final Weight Loss about consuming a healthy diet and eating small meals, let me explain:

Cathie told me that I needed to temporarily throw the scale away and carb-load within 24 hours of all long-distance runs 10 miles or longer. The purpose of carb-loading is to prevent bonking, which occurs when a person depletes the glycogen stores in their liver and muscles. When one bonks, the result is immediate fatigue coupled with the feeling of a total loss of energy. Bonking is largely preventable by ingesting enough carbs before strenuous exercise to ensure that the glycogen levels are sufficient. When performing vigorous exercise, people should have a substantial amount of stored muscle glycogen because it is the body's easiest and most efficient source of accessible energy.

This is why I am vehemently opposed to severely limiting carbs as part of a weight-loss program—you must have carbs in order to do any meaningful form of exercise. Cathie assured me that I would burn off all of the excess calories I ingested during my long-distance training runs. This was accurate advice and I continued to lose weight while I was training.

For the record, I accidentally bonked on two of my short midweek maintenance runs. The first time was during a three-mile run. I was running fine and suddenly became exhausted and had no energy—I felt like I was getting the crap kicked out of me with each stride. I had eaten part of a "power muffin" in the morning for breakfast and a broccoli salad for lunch and was running with very few carbs in my system. I managed to get through the run, however, it was grueling and I vowed never to make the same mistake again. The road to hell being paved with good intentions, I made the same mistake again a month and a half later on a four-mile maintenance run. Once again, I got through it, laughing at my misery during the entire last part of the run. I deserved my misery for making the same mistake twice. Fortunately, I never bonked on any of my long-distance training runs and I sure as hell was not going to risk bonking during the marathon.

My pre-marathon food fest was on and I continued to take full advantage of the situation. I needed to eat an 80/20 carb to protein ratio and not worry about the fat and the sugar I was ingesting in the process. I knew I would burn off all of the calories during the marathon, assuming I finished. Lunch was delicious; however, eating large quantities of carbs, sugar, and fat did not give me the same feeling of indulgence that it used to when I was living an unhealthy lifestyle. Following lunch, I took a short walk with Lisa and then went to the room for a much needed nap. I ate another big meal that evening for dinner: cream of mushroom soup, free range chicken with a side of gravy, and three rolls with butter.

Saturday, the day before the marathon, we woke up and I attacked the breakfast buffet at the hotel by eating five large pancakes drenched in butter and maple syrup, two hard-boiled eggs, yogurt, a few strips of bacon, and some green tea. I was eating like my old self again (except for the green tea). Following breakfast, we went to the hotel lobby and hired a taxi to tour the marathon route. Cathie advised me to tour the route in order to have a better mental image of the course.

Our taxi driver was an 80-year-old Japanese gentleman named Douglas. When Douglas was 10, he was living in Honolulu when Pearl Harbor was bombed. While we were in the taxi touring the marathon route, we listened to Douglas tell stories about watching the planes dropping bombs on Honolulu. It was a miracle that he had survived. The marathon course looked like I had imagined it would, however, it was hard to concentrate on the layout because I was fixated on Douglas and the stories he was sharing with us. The taxi ride with Douglas turned out to be one of the highlights of our Honolulu Marathon experience.

We returned to the hotel late in the morning and I took a nap. Per Cathie's instructions, I was not allowed to walk on the beach, go in the ocean, or sit in the Jacuzzi the day before the marathon. Walking in soft sand on the beach would put too much stress on my feet and ankles. Knowing I would be torturing them on race day, she wanted me to preserve them as much as possible. Going in the ocean or Jacuzzi would dehydrate me. I was also ordered to stay out of the sun as much as possible, which was easy since it was surprisingly cold, rainy, and windy most of the time we were in Honolulu.

I returned to the beach restaurant for a late lunch after my nap—eating exactly the same meal as I had eaten the day before (including a hot fudge sundae for dessert). I was concerned that I might be overdoing it on the food; however, I was about to run 26.2 miles and I knew that if I did not eat enough or under-carbed, I would be ruined on the course.

Following lunch, I enjoyed a half-mile slow jog. The jog was nothing more than an easy warm-up for the marathon the following morning. I had not run since Wednesday and needed to take myself through running strides and get my muscle memory juices flowing in preparation for the marathon. I was definitely on food overload and felt like I was running with a lead balloon in my stomach after everything I had eaten.

We planned to make it an early evening because we were waking up at 2:30 the following morning. The Honolulu Marathon official start time was 5 AM. Lisa and I went to the hotel room, opened my race packet, and removed my timing chip and zip ties. The most important item in my race packet was the timing chip. The timing chip is fixed on top of the shoelace on either the left or right running shoe and is attached using plastic ties. For additional peace of mind, the chip can be interlaced through the shoe lace. I was not about to try to secure the chip myself. If there is anyone who could screw that one up, it would be me. My civil engineer wife quickly figured it out and affixed the timing chip to my shoelace.

The timing chip allows sensors to record the time you cross the start line, your interval times during the race, and your finish time. One of the Honolulu Marathon rules was stated in bold print on the pre-race packet—no timing chip—no official credit for running or finishing the marathon.

Once my timing chip was fixed on top of my right running shoe and Lisa had assured me that only a stick of dynamite could remove it, I placed everything else that I would need for the marathon in its own separate bag including my race packet with my official marathon number (7314), the clothes I would wear, my Garmin, iPod, ear buds, goo packs, and shot bloks (shot bloks are small square-shaped energy sources that replenish carbohydrates and electrolytes in your body—similar to goo packs). I triple-checked everything down to the last detail. Once I knew I had everything ready to go, I was able enjoy the rest of the evening.

We walked down to Kapiolani Park where the finish line was located and picked a spot just beyond it where Lisa would hopefully be able to video me with her iPhone when I completed the race. Knowing we might not be able to meet in that exact place (there would be approximately 50,000 people in the park on race day), we chose a couple of back-up meeting places. One was near a small statue and the other was the tent where I would hopefully be picking up my finisher t-shirt.

Walking to Kapiolani Park the evening before the marathon was very relaxing. Lisa took photos of me pretending to run across the finish line. Her calm demeanor helped me relax and not think about the what ifs (what if I got a debilitating cramp and couldn't finish, what if I got injured, what if this was as crazy as many had thought when I first said I was going to run a marathon back in July, etc.). While we were at the park, I thought about how earlier in the year I was a completely out-of-shape obese person who weighed 271 pounds and had a 44-inch waist. I had been unable to walk on the treadmill at the gym without putting Vaseline on the insides of my legs to prevent them from chaffing. Now I was in Honolulu and in less than 24 hours I would be attempting to run a 26.2 mile marathon.

We stood at the finish line talking, laughing, and taking pictures. I weighed 194 pounds and had a size 33/34 waist. I could not believe how far I had come in such a short time. I was one day away from finally being able to know with conviction that I had traveled to the opposite side of the universe from being an obese, out-of-shape, highly processed-food-addicted overeater.

We walked away from the park that evening toward our hotel on Kalakaua Avenue. The beach was on our left and the shops were on the right side of the street. We had not made it half way back to the hotel when the rain began to pour down. The weather in Honolulu had been overcast since we had arrived. If we had been there exclusively for a vacation, I would have been bitterly disappointed. Since I was there to run a marathon, I was relieved to see the rain, overcast skies, and feel the persistent breeze. I hoped it would last one more day so that I would not be running any part of the marathon under a blistering hot sun.

It was time for me to have a world class pre-marathon dinner. I was not hungry at all. How could I be? During the last day and a half, I had eaten more than I normally would during a four-day stretch. The rain continued to hammer down and everyone on the street including us took cover in the shops on Kalakaua Avenue. We walked into the Hyatt Regency Waikiki Beach Hotel to get a restaurant recommendation. The concierge at the hotel recommended Hy's Steakhouse—just a few blocks away. It was dark and the rain dumped on us during our short walk to Hy's. Lisa and I were wearing shorts, t-shirts, sports jackets, and tennis shoes. Our clothes were soaked when we arrived.

Hy's Steakhouse is located on a non-descript walkway among various buildings and condominiums in Waikiki. You can't get a feel for what kind of place it is until you actually walk in the door. When we walked in, we saw that the two male employees at the host stand were wearing tuxedos and the hostess was elegantly dressed in a business suit, stockings, and high heels. The look on their faces when they saw us was priceless. I could tell they were 50/50 on whether we were street drunks or just low-rent tourists who showed up to ask for directions to the nearest ABC Souvenir Store. Recognizing this, I immediately informed them that their restaurant had been very highly recommended by the hotel concierge. With their most forced smiles of the evening they informed us that there wasn't any available seating in the restaurant.

We were told that we might be able to find seats at the bar at the back of the restaurant. As luck would have it, there were two seats at the end of the bar. This worked out perfectly—we would be eating dinner away from the other patrons who were much more elegantly dressed than we were. Since Lisa was not running in the marathon the following day, she took full advantage of the menu and ordered the famous Hy's rack of lamb, a Grey Goose Cosmo, and a cappuccino truffle for dessert. I ordered the Scampi Sicilian, which was the only pasta dish on the menu. I was not hungry but I knew I needed to keep carb loading. I ate like there was no tomorrow because I knew if I didn't there would be no tomorrow.

Earlier I described how people overeat at steakhouses. Case in point— the first item that Hy's Steakhouse serves before you order is a basket of piping hot cheese bread. I was all over the cheese bread. One basket of Hy's cheese bread could prevent someone from bonking in an ultramarathon. Lisa enjoyed one piece and I ate the other four. When our entrées arrived, I forced myself to eat more food.

I ate most of my pasta and a couple of pieces of shrimp that were probably sautéed in ten gallons of butter and oil. The food was well prepared and the cheese bread was to die for (both figuratively and literally). Lisa thoroughly enjoyed her lamb.

I politely requested a to-go box for the pasta only. The bartender (and waiter for the severely underdressed) looked at me like I was insane. He inquired as to why I was getting the pasta to go and throwing away all of the shrimp. When we informed him that I would be running the marathon the next morning, he looked at us for the first time like we were semi-respectable people. The dessert arrived and Lisa swears to this day that Hy's cappuccino truffle is one of the very best desserts that she has ever eaten. Lisa is a food snob, especially when it comes to dessert, so this is a compliment of the highest honor. I had a couple of bites of her dessert and it seemed fantastic; however, I was already slipping in and out of a food coma.

We walked past the host stand and exchanged goodbyes with the three hosts who had greeted us so warmly when we arrived. Their "thank you and have a nice evening" had the sincerity of "how is your day going" from a computer tech support person in Mumbai. The monsoon had slowed to a soft drizzle and our walk back to our hotel was uneventful.

When we arrived at the hotel, I retrieved my marathon race number from my race packet and Lisa attached it to my shirt. We meticulously laid everything out that I planned to use during the marathon so that I would not forget anything.

I was sound asleep by 10:00 PM. Four and a half hours later I woke up to the simultaneous sounds of the wake-up call from the hotel, Lisa's cell phone alarm clock, and the bedside alarm clock. I was excited. I put on my Nike shirt, Brooks running shorts, and New Balance running shoes. I never heard from the sponsors from any of these companies—they must have accidentally misplaced my number.

I placed three goo packs in the pockets of my running shorts and three shot blocks wrapped in clear plastic wrap on the inside ankle portion of each running sock. I clipped my iPod to the bottom of my shirt (after checking to make sure it had charged), taped the earbud cord to the inside of my shirt, ate a few handfuls of left-over pasta from the steakhouse, grabbed a bottle of water to drink on the bus, kissed Lisa, and left the hotel.

I walked in a crowd down Kalakaua Avenue at 3:15 and boarded a bus at the Honolulu Zoo to join more than 20,000 other people at the marathon starting line.

Following a 10-minute ride, the bus arrived at Ala Moana Beach Park. I walked a short distance through the park to the starting area. I could not believe that I was standing in a crowd of people this large at 4 in the morning. The energy was electrifying and the marathon would not start for another hour!

I discovered that when you run in a marathon that has thousands of runners, you are "corralled" behind the starting line with groups of people according to your anticipated finishing time. The "frontrunners" (Kenyans, Ethiopians, and superior marathon runners who would finish the marathon, give interviews, eat breakfast, and watch a pay per view movie back at their hotel rooms by the time I crossed the finish line) were at the very front of the start line. All others were grouped behind them according to their anticipated finishing time. I hoped to finish the marathon in a little over five hours so I placed myself in the group that was in the five to six hour area.

Five AM arrived and the runners at the front of the line who I never saw at any point during the race were off. I enjoyed the beautiful fireworks display that officially started the marathon while slowly moving forward toward the start line. I crossed the start line at approximately 5:12, started my Garmin timer, and I was off. I was officially running in a marathon. The first two miles I maneuvered around people who were moving very slowly, even walking. I was not bothered by this because all I could think about was the fact that I was finally running in the marathon that had been the subject of conversation of everyone in my immediate circle of family and friends for the last four months.

I felt sufficiently humble and very excited all at the same time. I estimated that between 6 and 6:30 I would be running past the hotel where Lisa and I were staying. We had not specifically planned for her to be standing out on the curb in front of our hotel because we had no idea what the crowd situation would be. Lisa had stayed up with me until I left the room. The hotel was on the right side of the street where I would be running. Although it was still dark, there was enough lighting from the street lamps for me to look for her ahead of time. When I was about 20 yards away from the hotel, I saw her standing on the edge of the curb recording me with her iPhone. Seeing her there meant the world to me. Always thinking ahead, she even brought me an extra goo pack. While running past, I slowed down, took the goo pack, stole a kiss, and kept running.

The goo pack she gave me is the first one that I used during the race. I consumed it just before I started the trek up Diamond Head Road once I reached the end of Kapiolani Park. I thoroughly enjoyed the first part of the marathon. I high-fived spectators and gave race photographers my best "this is fun and no big deal smile" as I ran past. The Honolulu Marathon organizers had photographers stationed at nine places throughout the marathon course. They were easy to spot because there was a large "smile sign" on the side of the road that alerted you to the fact that you were about to have your picture taken.

I completed the run up Diamond Head road and reached mile 10. I passed Kapiolani Community College and was on Kilauea Avenue headed toward Kalanianaole Highway. I settled into running the marathon, and the uniqueness of the experience started to wear off. The marathon had become another long training run. A little nugget that I picked up in a running magazine suggested viewing a marathon as a number of mileage laps rather than a 26.2 mile run in order to make the distance not seem so arduous. The way I mentally arranged my laps was the first 6.2 miles would be lap one, which would leave me with four remaining five-mile laps. I passed mile 11 and entered Kalanianaole Highway. In my mind, I was beginning the third lap of a five-lap run. This worked very well for me because I usually started feeling stiff and sore when I crossed 12 miles on my long runs. I was mentally on lap three of five and had already completed a good part of the race.

While running up Kalanianaole Highway on miles 11-15 on one side, you see the faster runners on the other side of the highway running miles 18-22. I felt like I was closer to the back of the group of all of the marathon runners than I really was—especially considering that I made my one and only bathroom stop and waited in an eight minute line at the portable toilets. When I started running again, I passed many runners who had stopped to work out cramps, rest, or quit altogether.

I ran past mile marker 15, exited the highway on Hawaii Kai Drive, and circled around a loop on Keahole Street, re-entering the highway half-way through the 17th mile. I was now headed in the opposite direction where I had been running in miles 11-15. Mentally, I was running back toward the finish line. There were many local residents standing out on the street cheering us on, handing out cold wet sponges, water, and Gatorade, and holding up inspirational signs throughout the race. I made eye contact with many people who made eye contact with me while I was running. Hawaiians are wonderful, gracious people.

Despite their support, I was feeling the effects of how far I had run. As I approached mile marker 18, I could see all of the runners on the other side of the highway that had yet to make the loop at mile marker 15. I could not believe there were that many people so far behind me! I was intrigued by this and focused on them as much as possible because I was trying not to think about how much my body was starting to hurt.

There were many runners who looked much fitter than me who were running behind me in the marathon. This intrigued me. I had managed to acquire a little "cut definition" on my frame (particularly in my legs) and otherwise looked like a reasonably healthy 5'10" middle-aged man. Many of the runners I could see who were running behind me appeared to be extremely fit and looked as though they had never carried even a moderate amount of body fat on their frame.

I was able to focus on this and ignore my pain until I had almost reached the 20th mile. When I got to mile 20, I was in a significant amount of pain and only thinking about trying to finish the race. My rib cage hurt, my quads and hips were sore, and my legs and ankles felt like someone had hit them with a baseball bat. Thankfully, the goo packs and shot blocks I consumed had prevented me from cramping, but I was out of goo packs and only had one shot block left.

I remembered people telling me that the marathon is two segments— the first 20 miles and the last 6.2 miles. A guy in my gym actually told me that the marathon does not really start until you cross mile marker 20 and begin running the last 6.2 miles. I brought this up to Cathie before I left. She advised me not to borrow trouble and pre-suppose what bad things might happen during the race.

When I crossed mile marker 20, a pebble kicked up into my left shoe. With each stride I felt like I was being stabbed with a dull knife in the bottom of my left foot. I tried to block it out and keep running but it hurt too much. To say that I was pissed off at this point would be putting it mildly. The last thing I needed was anything else to contend with including another challenge, or another form of pain in addition to the pain I was already feeling. I saw a concrete wall on the side of the highway road and decided to run over to it, lean against it, and dump out my shoe. When I stepped up on the curb having just run over 20 miles, I felt like I had just climbed a mountain. While dumping the pebble out my shoe and cursing my bad luck, my conversation with the lady in the Starbucks line at the Portland airport popped into my head. I had run the last three miles consumed with how badly my body was hurting and kept wondering if I would be able to hold up long enough to cross the finish line.

The remainder of the race would be different because I arrived at the following conclusion: I am in Hawaii and of all things I am running a marathon! I just crossed mile 20—six more miles and this will all be over. I will never get to live my first and perhaps only marathon experience ever again. From this moment on I will be in the moment and enjoy the rest of this incredible adventure. I will make eye contact with all of the wonderful, gracious people on the side of the road who have come out to support the marathon runners. I will run the entire rest of the marathon with a smile on my face regardless of my pain.

With that in mind and the pebble out of my shoe, I gingerly stepped off the curb and started running again. Just before mile marker 22, I exited Kalanianaole Highway onto Kealaolu Avenue and was running through neighborhoods. There were so many residents standing out in the street handing out sponges, water, and Gatorade.

I specifically remember running past other racers and gaining momentum as I entered Kahala Avenue from Kealaolu Avenue. I was not thinking about my pain or worrying about finishing the marathon. I was completely in the moment—just like the lady in the Starbucks line told me to be. This was the last piece of the puzzle that would enable me to achieve something that I never could have dreamed possible seven and a half months before.

My next memory of running in the marathon was running down Diamond Head Road and seeing mile marker 25. Just before that mile marker, there was a sign that read, "2.2 kilometers left. You are going to make it." I felt both sweat and tears running down my face as I ran.

I reached the bottom of Diamond Head Road and saw Kapiolani Park. I felt complete euphoria and realized my moment was about to arrive. The sun was out, the park was crowded, and I was about to make the last turn on to Kalakaua Avenue. In a short distance I would be viewing the finish line.

When I turned onto Kalakaua Avenue, I was running faster than I had the entire marathon. There were so many people in the park (estimated 50,000) cheering and screaming words of encouragement to all of the marathon runners. The energy and the excitement of the moment inspired me to continue to run faster as I approached the finish line. I passed so many other runners during the final stretch of the marathon. Passing other runners during the final stretch of the marathon made me feel like I was finishing the race strong, which was important to me. Although my body would not have appreciated it, I could have run further had I needed to. I didn't need to run any further—I crossed the finish line with an official time of 5:15:23.

I entered the finisher area and saw a policeman standing between the crowd and the runners who were just crossing the finish line. He had an ear-to ear-grin and directed us to continue walking through the finish area. I looked for Lisa immediately as I crossed the finish line. Although she was not in our chosen meeting spot, I knew I would find her at one of our back-up meeting places in the park. The first time I stopped moving in the finish area was in front of one of the volunteers so she could place a shell lei around my neck. My next stop was the outdoor showers which were spewing cold water. I joined the other finishers and walked under the shower heads. When I walked through the outdoor shower, it occurred to me that I should turn off the timer on my Garmin.

There is a short (though it didn't seem short at the time) path that led from the showers into Kapiolani Park. I was blown away by all of the people standing on either side of the path smiling and congratulating us as we walked into the park. I cannot adequately put into words the euphoria I felt. I entered the park on a mission to find Lisa and share the moment with her. I searched for our second meeting place, which was next to a statue by a pond. I could not find it—how typical!

Meeting place three was the tent where the marathon finishers were awarded t-shirts. Lisa found me walking to the finisher tent and we finally were able to share a warm embrace. This was the culmination of all of the life-changing events that had transpired since I began my final weight loss back in April. Lisa took a picture of me wearing my size L finisher t-shirt on her iPhone and posted it on Facebook. She texted the same picture to Cathie.

Lisa informed me that my cell phone and Facebook page were already blowing up with congratulatory messages. Technology is amazing. The Honolulu Marathon website updated times and splits throughout the race and immediately posted finishing times. A few of my close friends had been tracking my progress throughout the marathon and knew my exact finishing time before I did!

There were 19,078 participants who finished the Honolulu marathon that day. The average finish time was 5:55:46. My finish time of 5:15:23 put me in 6,892nd place—well into the top 40% of all finishers. Every conceivable goal related to running a marathon that I had set for myself had been accomplished.

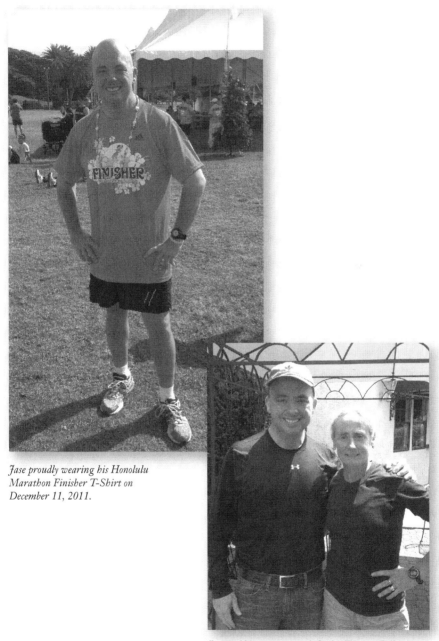

Jase proudly wearing his Honolulu Marathon Finisher T-Shirt on December 11, 2011.

Jase and his running coach Cathie Twomey Bellamy.

Chapter TWELVE

A CHANGED LIFE

When you commit to taking back your life, many opportunities become available to you that would never have been possible as an overweight or obese person—for me, the Honolulu Marathon was only the beginning. When Lisa and I returned home, I could not have imagined all of the events during the next month that would reinforce the difference my weight loss would make.

We had just launched Cheval Amour two days before leaving. Cheval Amour is an equestrian-inspired clothing brand that Lisa conceptualized, created, and runs full time in addition to her civil-engineering consulting practice. Lisa has ridden horses since before she could walk. Horses are her passion, and being an avid equestrian inspired Lisa to launch a beautiful and environmentally responsible line of clothing. I could not be more proud. View the online store at **www.chevalamour.com.**

I could not wait to talk to my coach and now good friend, Cathie Twomey Bellamy. Cathie left a message on my cell phone Sunday evening after she received the picture of me wearing my finisher t-shirt sent from Lisa's iPhone. When I listened to Cathie's message, I realized how emotionally invested she had been in me running the marathon.

Lisa and I enjoyed a celebratory dinner with Cathie and her husband, Ron the week we arrived home. I could not wait to thank her in person. Cathie engineered a wishful pipe dream into a stunning reality that I will appreciate and cherish for the rest of my life. We agreed (Cathie told me and I agreed) during dinner that evening that I would be taking the next month off from serious running and training. My body needed to heal. Additionally, she wanted me to enjoy some mental downtime before deciding what my next goal would be. I can't imagine why Cathie thought I might make a rash decision related to running!

I flew to San Francisco the following morning to attend business meetings for the next few days. I had the entire first day to do as I wished because my meetings would not begin until the following day. Saturday, December 17, was a spectacular day in San Francisco. I considered playing golf but decided to walk down to the bay from my hotel instead. I walked from the top of Nob Hill down to Pier 39 where I had completed my favorite marathon training run only a month and a half earlier. When I reached Pier 39, I could not resist firing up my iPod and taking off on a relaxing "fun run." I ran through Crissy Field, up the paths, and crossed the Golden Gate Bridge. I sat at Golden Gate Vista Point on the north side of the bridge in Sausalito for an hour enjoying the 75-degree sunny day while reflecting on everything that had transpired during the previous months. It had been only six days since I had run the marathon in Honolulu and I had just trekked from the top of Nob Hill to the north side of the Golden Gate Bridge. I was enjoying a perfect day outside in one of the most beautiful cities in the world. My outlook on life had changed dramatically in every regard. I walked/ran over ten miles that day and could not have enjoyed it more.

I returned home to Eugene to enjoy the Christmas holidays and ring in the New Year with family and friends. Despite all of the celebrating I did over the holidays, I continued to eat healthfully prepared foods (including sweets), drink plenty of water, and exercise. January 1, 2012, I weighed 188 pounds!

The first week of the New Year I flew to Dallas to visit two of my long-time close friends—Jeffrey, whom I have known since childhood, and Richard, whom I have known since college. Although they were both aware of my weight loss and successful marathon run, I had not seen either one of them since I started losing weight. Their stunned reaction when they first saw me reminded me of how far I had come in a short period of time.

One morning while I was in Dallas, Jeffrey and I ventured out on a four-mile run. During our run, Jeffrey told me that if he had to guess at the beginning of the year 2011 which one of his friends he thought would have run a marathon by the end of the year, he would have picked me last. He could not believe how easy it was for me to run four miles. In many respects, I could not either. The last time I had seen him, I could not run four blocks.

I knew I was not through running. The thought of running another marathon did not appeal to me. I decided my next accomplishment would be to train for and run an ultramarathon, an athletic event that involves running any distance race that is greater than the length of a marathon. I laughed at what I could only imagine would be the look on Cathie's face when I returned home and informed her that I wanted to tackle an ultra. Time to go back to the coffee shop and have another discussion! Poor woman, what did she ever do to deserve this?

While I was in Dallas, I was contacted by Randi Bjornstad from The Register-Guard newspaper. She had heard about my weight loss and successful marathon run and wanted to interview me and write a story about it.

I returned late Tuesday evening on January 10, 2012. The following afternoon I sat in a conference room for two hours at the newspaper discussing the events that had taken place related to my weight loss, marathon training, and running the Honolulu Marathon. Had it really only been eight and a half months? The day I was interviewed, I weighed 185 pounds—nine pounds less than I weighed when I ran the Honolulu Marathon.

Randi told me at the end of our meeting that my article would appear in the newspaper on Monday, January 16. I imagined the article would be two or three paragraphs buried on the fifth or sixth page of some section of the paper. I hoped that there would be a few people who desperately needed to lose weight who would find the article and follow in my footsteps.

Rather than being focused on the upcoming article, I was looking forward to getting together with Cathie to discuss training for my first ultramarathon. The one I wanted to run was on April 22, 2012. Finishing an ultramarathon on April 22 would be an extraordinary accomplishment because it would mean that I would have run a marathon and an ultramarathon within a year of starting my life-changing weight loss.

Cathie and I decided to meet Monday, the day the article would appear. I woke up on Monday at 7 AM and my cell phone was buzzing with congratulatory text messages from people who had already read the article. I was surprised by this because I could not believe that people were awake and had found the article about me buried somewhere in the newspaper. When I arrived at Starbucks in Eugene to meet Cathie, I saw the newspaper for the first time and was stunned. There was a large picture of me running in the Honolulu Marathon splashed across the front page of the Life Section accompanied by a one-and-a-half-page article!

My email address was included in the article. I received congratulatory emails from people in Oregon, Idaho, and Washington for the next few weeks. Most were people I had never met. Many asked for weight-loss advice. I responded to every email I received and was invited to speak to a weight-loss group in Portland.

February 1, 2012, weighing 181 pounds, I gave my first motivational talk and shared my story with a group of about 30 people who were looking for sound weight-loss advice from someone they could identify with. I had been in their shoes only eight months earlier. The response was overwhelming. That evening I became convinced that sharing my personal story could help many others who no longer wished to live a compromised life due to a weight problem.

Final Weight-Loss Lesson

The Setback

Setbacks can and will occur during your life (usually at the most inconvenient time) whether you are trying to lose weight or not. Although it sounds like a cliché, it is what you do in response to a setback that determines your personal success or failure. My setback occurred on February 13 at McCarran Airport in Las Vegas.

The ultramarathon was a little over two months away and I had just completed an 18-mile training run in Las Vegas two days prior on February 11. My running route included significant elevation changes that were similar to the ultramarathon I was planning to run on April 22. The day after I ran 18 miles, I played golf. I could not have had a better time even though my golf game officially sucked due to a combination of factors including my new swing, lack of play, and the fact that I although I enjoy golf immensely, I'm not very good.

Monday morning I was walking toward the security line at the airport when in an instant the right side of my body from my lower back down to my ankle was suddenly in excruciating pain. I could not imagine what was wrong with me. I made it through the hellish security line and limped into a convenience shop and immediately took four Advil. I knew my two-hour flight back to Eugene was going to be miserable—and miserable was an understatement. The Advil I took did not begin to tackle the pain that I was feeling—it was like putting a Snoopy Band-Aid on a ruptured carotid artery. Lisa picked me up from the airport and drove me straight home. I could not sit in the passenger seat for most of the ride—I had to kneel in the seat facing backward because it was too painful to sit.

I visited my primary care physician and Robert, my physical therapist, that week. Once it was determined that I could not execute a heel raise using my right leg or even feel myself trying to raise my heel, I was immediately scheduled to have my first MRI. The MRI revealed that I had a herniated L-5 S-1 disc. Tuesday, March 6 I met with a neurosurgeon. After reviewing my MRI, he determined that the only option that made sense was for me to undergo surgery immediately to correct the problem. He explained that the herniation could have been caused by any number of things throughout my life (I am fairly certain that carrying an extra 90-100 pounds around for years might have been a factor). He assured me that there had not been a specific event that caused the disc herniation. I was not lifting weights or engaging in any kind of serious physical exercise during the onset of my pain, I was slowly walking through an airport. All surgeries are a big deal, particularly surgeries involving the back and spine. Prior to my surgery I reached out to friends in the medical community and was assured that the surgical procedure to correct my disc herniation would be minimally invasive and not particularly dangerous as far as surgeries go.

I realized the ultramarathon I was planning to run on April 22 was not going to happen for me. I had anticipated that the last chapter of this book would be about my finishing an ultramarathon in April in addition to finishing the Honolulu Marathon back in December. Both events would have occurred before the one-year anniversary of my life-changing weight loss. Instead, my injury gave me another example of how much my perspective on life had changed as a result of my weight loss.

I had a very successful surgery on March 13, and was able to walk out of the surgery center a few hours after my procedure because I was in premium physical condition. Had I gone into surgery weighing 271 pounds, the surgery would have been much more difficult and my recovery would have been prolonged and miserable. I experienced minimal pain and discomfort during the week following my surgery.

I returned to my neurosurgeon's office a week after my surgery for a post-op check-up and was informed that I would not be able to engage in any exercise other than walking on a treadmill for two months—no running, no strength training, and no cross-training. I was specifically instructed not to lift anything heavier than a gallon of milk. Having completed an 18-mile training run in preparation for an ultramarathon only a few weeks prior, I was not exactly thrilled that my only means of exercise for the next two months would be walking on a treadmill.

I returned home depressed and immediately went to our bedroom to lie down. Not only would I not be running the ultramarathon, I would have to suspend my exercise program for two months.

Exercise and running had become very important to me. I was extremely confident in my physical condition and mentally prepared to successfully complete an ultramarathon. I had easily accomplished everything that Cathie had asked of me prior to my injury, including the 18-mile training run in Las Vegas.

Cathie could not have been more supportive after she learned of my injury. When I told her that my only form of exercise would be walking for two months, she informed me that the moment I stepped on the treadmill, I was back in training. This was exactly what I needed to hear.

I walked on various treadmills for five to seven hours each week for two months and engaged in no other exercise—no strength training, no gym cardio, and no running. I missed strenuous exercise terribly and could not wait to resume.

Final Weight-Loss Lesson
My back injury was a setback—nothing more, nothing less. The formerly obese Jase Simmons would have reacted to this unfortunate situation by reverting to an unhealthy lifestyle that would have included eliminating exercising altogether, consuming an unhealthy diet, and gaining weight. The thought of pulling that crap never crossed my mind this time. I walked for exercise, continued to eat healthfully prepared, minimally processed and unprocessed foods, and drank substantial amounts of water—all core principles of my permanent healthy-eating program.

I went into surgery on the morning of March 13, weighing 181 pounds. During the two months following my operation, I stayed on my healthy-eating program, exercised by walking on a treadmill, and lost another 13 pounds! This should tell you everything you need to know about how important it is to consume a healthy diet that consists of minimally processed and unprocessed foods in the right macronutrient ratios. To be clear, I had lost 90 pounds prior to undergoing back surgery and then managed to lose another 13 pounds during the two months following my back surgery despite the fact that my only means of exercise was walking on a treadmill.

April 25, 2012

I weighed myself on the one-year-anniversary date of the beginning of my weight loss. The scale revealed that my weight was 176 pounds—I had lost 95 pounds in one year! My 27-year weight problem is behind me forever and I will never be overweight again. Not only do I have my quality of life back, I have the opportunity to educate and motivate others to successfully travel down a path toward their own Final Weight Loss.

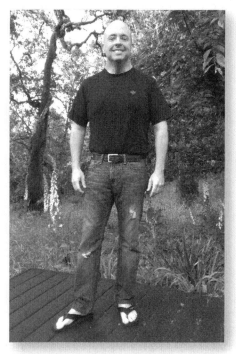

Jase a few days after celebrating his 44th birthday.

Postscript

After I ran the Honolulu Marathon, Cathie told me I would always be a runner. I resumed my 5-95 Weight-Loss Exercise Program two months after my back surgery and started running again. I currently offer private weight-loss coaching and counseling services to individuals and small groups. Additionally, I have launched a speaking business and look forward to giving motivational and informational speeches to groups and companies on the subject of health and weight loss. The greatest reward that I have received as a result of my own weight loss is the opportunity to help others reclaim their lives just like I have reclaimed mine. My weight currently fluctuates between 167 and 170 pounds—perhaps I have reached my optimum healthy weight. Only time will tell. I will never be overweight again.

Acknowledgements

Without the following people, none of what you have just read would have been possible:

To my late father and mother, Dr. and Mrs. James H. Simmons, who raised me to believe that anything is possible.

To my wife, Lisa Kelly Simmons, who supported me during many failed attempts at weight loss and gently encouraged me to keep trying until I finally got it right, always loving me unconditionally.

To my in-laws, Jeffrey and Katherine Kelly, who selflessly spent countless hours reading, advising, and editing my work.

To my sister-in-law, Shawna Kelly, who selflessly spent countless hours reading, advising, and editing my work.

To my editor Jill Kelly, who gave *Final Weight Loss* a comprehensive clean edit and patiently guided me through the remaining challenging stages of turning a manuscript into a published book (www.jillkellyeditor.com).

To Sarah Bertram, USAW Sports Performance Certified Personal Trainer, who provided me with extensive strength-training knowledge and effective circuit-training workouts that anyone following my program will benefit from for years to come.

To Melinda Clark, LMT, who is truly gifted and passionate about her craft. Melinda's professional therapeutic massage and bodywork consistently enables me to recover from strenuous exercise and long training runs each week.

To Robert Wayner, PT, for creating the RunWell Program, healing my physical injuries, and improving my gait cycle. Without Robert, I would have never made it to the start line in Honolulu.

To Cathie Twomey Bellamy, whose extensive knowledge as a running coach and world-class athlete made it possible for a novice runner like me to fulfill a dream that was far beyond what should have been attainable. I still owe you that 5K!

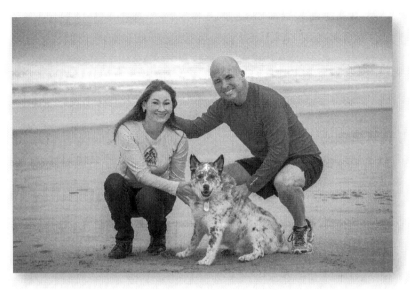

Jase, Lisa, and Kodi having fun on the Oregon Coast.

Jase Simmons lives in Creswell, Oregon, with his wife Lisa and various four-legged animals they call their children. Jase counsels groups and individuals on weight loss and shares his inspiring story by giving motivational speeches.

For more information about Jase, visit
www.weightlossjase.com.

Jase writes a weight-loss blog at
www.weightlossjase.blogspot.com.

Contact him directly at
weightlossjase@gmail.com.

17691695R00099

Made in the USA
Charleston, SC
23 February 2013